Intermittent Fasting And Ketogenic Diet Bible

Reset Your Metabolism With The Keto Diet, Fast Your Way To A Flat Belly, Increase Longevity, And Experience The Life-changing Benefits Of Keto Clarity

Diana Monroe

Table of Contents

Introduction

This book will inform you about the intermittent fasting and ketogenic diets. You may want to use these diet plans separately or combine them for maximum weight loss benefits. The keto diet and the intermittent fasting diet are quite popular for weight loss, building muscle, and boosting one's energy levels. Combining these methods will help you achieve better results, however, you can choose only one if that's your preference.

In this book, you will learn all you need to know about these two diets, the foods to eat, as well as sample recipes that you may want to try out. Don't even try to put this book down because you are only pages away from finding out the best methods in weight loss and health gains!

Chapter One: Introduction To Intermittent Fasting

What is Intermittent Fasting?

Intermittent fasting is one of the most popular trends in the world's health and fitness arena. Numerous studies have revealed that this meal plan has great effects on our body and brain, it's even capable of prolonging your lifespan. Intermittent fasting is the type of fasting where one divides their time into eating periods and fasting periods. For instance, you could have your day set up so that you can eat any time between noon and eight p.m. When the period to eat ends, that is eight p.m. onwards, you refrain from eating until the next day at noon. It's as simple as that.

In actuality, intermittent fasting is not a diet but an eating pattern. This eating plan does not tell you what to eat but rather when to eat. A lot of people have no idea that while they are asleep, they are actually on a fasting period. You can lengthen the fasting phase by forfeiting breakfast and having your first meal at midday (your "break-fast" meal), and your last meal of the day at eight in the night.

The most popular kind of fasting plan involves fasting for sixteen hours a day and having an eight-hour window for feeding. While no food is allowed during the fasting period, you may have non-caloric beverages like water or tea.

There is this common question that people ask; how frequently should I fast? This is a personal decision and it varies from person to person. Some do it every week while others take longer breaks. There is no wrong way of fasting. You just need to listen to how your body responds to a fasting plan to learn what's best for you.

Intermittent fasting is practiced for different reasons, losing weight and improving your overall health are the ones we're interested in in this book. Unlike other forms of dieting that limit the kind and amount of food you eat, intermittent fasting focuses on the time of eating. You don'☐t necessarily have to change your diet. You can have whichever foods you would like to eat as long as it is in the time frame you set for eating.

Fasting has been practiced since ancient human times and it used to be out of necessity. In the past, food was more scarce, and without technology, availability was subject to the time of year. As a result, our ancestors had to go without food for long periods. Fasting is also practiced across several ancient religions like Islam, Christianity, Judaism, and Buddhism.

When people fast by choice perhaps it's because it creates changes on a cellular and molecular level. Your hormone levels adjust to make your body fats more accessible. Additionally, your cells also initiate processes of repair and alter gene expressions. When you fast, some of these things are affected:

- The human growth hormone: their levels increase almost five times and are beneficial in losing fat and building muscles, among other positive changes.

- Insulin: insulin levels drop and sensitivity to it improves. Lower levels of insulin make it easier for stored body fats to be accessed.
- Cell repair: each time you fast, your body begins the cell repairing process. This happens when cells get rid of old and dysfunctional proteins that build up within the cells.
- Expression of genes: changes occur in the gene functions that relate to long life and protection against illnesses.

Why Fast?

People may decide to fast for many reasons:

• One may fast as a way of practicing their spirituality: either to cleanse their souls, or to increase patience, or as a sacrifice during a holy period.

• To lose weight: people may be fasting to reduce their weight.

• To better their health: It has been documented that fasting can improve the overall health of an individual.

If you would like to know how to helpfully and safely get on a fasting regime, this is the book for you. Find out everything you need to know about intermittent fasting; from clearly outlined steps on how to do it, to the benefits awaiting you. You will get to know the different types of intermittent fasting and choose one that suits you. This is a great guide for your fasting journey, including after you start fasting, with information on how to exercise and eat well and stay motivated throughout the fasting period.

I hope that you will enjoy reading this book and getting the insights that will help you with intermittent fasting. Have an insightful read!

The History of Intermittent Fasting

Compared to traditional diets, fasting is simple and well-defined. Unknowingly, a majority of us already practice intermittent fasting when we skip meals such as breakfast or dinner. During the days of hunting and gathering, our forefathers always fasted when they were low on their supply of food.

After agriculture came into existence, what followed was a more recognizably modern civilization. Whole cities as well as great castles stored grain and preserved meat for the winter season. However, when there was a scarcity of food due to changing seasons, fasting was often required. Before people used irrigation, inadequate rainfall meant famine. As a result, the population fasted to make their food supply last longer until a point when the rains would resume and make it possible for the crops to do well again.

During this era, religions also prospered because of people living closely and sharing their ideas with each other. Many religious groups also recommended fasting. Hindus refer to fasting as Vaasa and it is observed during special occasions as a personal penance or as a way of honoring their gods. Islam and Judaism observe Ramadan and Yom Kippur, respectively. During these periods of fasting, believers are not allowed to engage in sexual activities, work, wash, or even wear leather. When it comes to Catholics, they fast six weeks before Easter.

The Science of Intermittent Fasting

Modernization has really changed the way we view and consume food on a day-to-day basis. This has also led to many health issues that our society faces. Even though intermittent fasting is an ancient practice, now is when many people are being enlightened as to its health benefits. When you practice fasting, what you do is to allow your body to naturally detoxify and repair itself. There are three main mechanisms of fasting that promote good health: circadian biology, lifestyle behaviors, and the gut microbiome.

Intermittent fasting is also easily accessible to just about everybody- compared to other diets, this one is simple. Many people's dieting resolutions are broken in just fourteen days. Dieting is about counting calories, reducing calories, as well as altering eating patterns. All of that involves extensive meal planning and preparation.

A majority of Americans go on diets every year but obesity is still a major national problem. It is evident that something is not working. With intermittent fasting, you don't need to painstakingly reduce your calorie intake by portioning every meal, but instead, the reduction naturally occurs through the limited feeding window. However, it is still recommended that you make an effort not to take in too many calories. This is a simple way of eating, a mere lifestyle change, that encourages loss of weight without affecting your lean tissue.

Chapter Summary

In this chapter, we discussed:

- What intermittent fasting is
- Reasons for intermittent fasting
- The history and science of intermittent fasting

In the next chapter, you will learn how to use intermittent fasting.

Chapter Two: How Intermittent Fasting Works

Exercise and Nutrition with Intermittent Fasting

We have already learned how easy it is to start intermittent fasting, you simply choose the feeding window that works for you! Once you start your intermittent fasting successfully, the next step is maintaining it, and making sure you're getting good results from it. Your diet, as well as your workout routine, may have to change to accommodate the fasting. Here□'s the best way to go about it.

Nutrition for Intermittent Fasting

One of the main reasons why people seem to be taking up intermittent fasting is that it doesn□'t restrict what one can eat. For some people, the idea of counting every single calorie that goes through their mouth is not very appealing.

Being able to lose weight, improve cognition and even maintain good blood sugar levels without restricting one'□s meals to a measly salad is very appealing. However, now that you aren'□t restricted to a specific type of food, does that mean you can eat whole tubs of ice cream when you're not fasting and live on nothing but fried foods?

If your aim is to lose weight, then, obviously, you won'□t get the best results in this way.

Because you're eating less you don't need to watch yourself as closely as you would on a normal diet. But if you want the full health benefits possible there are ways to maximize your eating time.

There are so many foods you can eat to improve your health and sustain your body for longer periods of time. We all know there are "good" and "bad" kinds of calories. Especially when fasting, you want food options that will help you take in the best kinds of calories for the limited time you eat. Some foods are meant to provide the full range of nutrients your body needs to be healthy, others, are specifically to help you feel fuller longer, you won't want to break your fast! Here are some things that should be in your meal rotation if they aren't already:

1. Water

This is one of the most important ingredients for body health, *and you should be drinking water even during your fasting period.* You want to keep your body hydrated especially because you□'re fasting. Water is also very vital for different body organs including the kidney and lungs.

The amount you take in may vary but try to take in as much water as you can. Drink water even after you have your last meal of the day as well as during your eating window. Water will help keep your belly full. If you do not like plain water or want to switch it up a bit, you can add a squeeze of lemon or some mint leaves to change the taste.

2. Vegetables

These include broccoli, kale, cauliflower, and Brussels sprouts. They are rich in vitamins, minerals, and fiber that you need for good health.

Avoid constipation by eating foods rich in fiber, regular bowel movements will help you feel and be healthy.

Other than that, fiber also contributes to the feeling of fullness, making your fast that much easier for you.

3. Legumes

You need the energy for everyday activities. Add carbs to your diet to give you energy during your fast, which can be any legume; beans, lentils, peas, black beans, and chickpeas are a few of the legumes you can add to your diet to keep you energized for the day.

4. Whole grains

Whole grain foods are rich in nutrients like fiber, Vitamin B, minerals and even antioxidants. Be sure to add whole grain foods to your meal plan. Some good options include brown rice, oatmeal, and sorghum.

5. Fish

You might have heard that fish is good for the brain. Other than making your brain more alert fish is also packed with fats, protein, and vitamin D. The richness of nutrients makes fish a great food for you when you are taking less food in throughout the day.

6. Fruits

These are a must-have for any diet, especially those rich in Vitamin C, including Kiwi, berries, citrus fruits like oranges, and papaya. Vitamin C tends to boost your immune system to keep you strong and less susceptible to diseases.

7. Eggs

These may be your source of protein while you go through your intermittent fasting. Remember that you want to build those muscles while getting rid of fat, which means that you need lots of protein. Plus, eggs are so easy to prepare. You can hard boil an egg for when you break your fast, scramble it, or make a quick and easy omelet (maybe throw in some of the veggies mentioned above) and move on with your day.

8. Avocado

The avocado works wonders to keep you fuller for longer. If you have been struggling with going for hours without a bite to eat then you should try adding just half an avocado with your lunch or dinner.

Distributing Nutrients in Your Meals

With this list of foods, you can now get a better idea of what you should be having during your eating period. You can distribute these types of foods into your different meals, making sure you have a bit of every nutrient when you eat.

Try to maintain a high-vegetable and protein intake through your eating period. It's best not to eat too much food all at once. Instead, have only enough to nourish your body, and last you to the next time you have to eat. Besides, eating a huge meal at lunchtime would probably make you uncomfortable while carrying out your other daily activities.

You should be having a combination of protein, vitamins, and healthy fats at a meal. For example, this could be a lunch of chicken, a leafy green salad, and half an avocado.

How to Incorporate the Right Exercises into Intermittent Fasting

Intermittent fasting may affect your workout routine if you have one. You will most likely be working with less energy because of your reduced caloric intake. This means you can'☐t keep up intense workouts while eating less- at least not in the first few days before your body gets used to fasting.

Shifting Your Workout Time

Depending on the type of fast you choose, you may need to change the time you exercise to a more convenient time.

For instance, if you decide on the 16/8 plan, you may not want to hit the gym early in the morning. The 16/8 fasting plan involves avoiding food and calorie-containing drinkings for sixteen hours but being allowed a window of eight hours to eat anything. You can repeat this cycle for as long as you wish. This usually means your first meal won't be until noon. So, in the morning you will be low on energy and won☐'t do as much as you would have done anyway.

Remember, intensely working out on no food can lead to lightheadedness or even fainting. You should consider moving your most intense workout sessions to within your eating period. This should leave you with enough energy to complete a regular routine.

You also have the option of changing your eating period so that your first meal of the day comes earlier, but your last meal would also shift back a few hours.

Reducing Your Workouts

If you have been exercising to lose fat, then you can ease up on the workouts when you start on intermittent fasting. Remember, fasting all on its own helps you to lose fat especially if coupled with a good diet. So, there may not be a need for excessive exercising.

Exercising on an Empty Stomach

You may decide to schedule your workout for just before you eat. Having a mild workout session before your eating window can actually have positive effects.

Normally, when you do some exercise, your body uses up glycogen, that is, the carbohydrates it has stored. However, when you are hungry, such as when your last meal was hours ago, you may not have enough carbs stored. This forces your body to dip into its stored fats to use for energy. This is how you get rid of fat to leave only muscle in your body.

There can be some drawbacks. Your body may also end up burning protein for energy, instead of fat, when there is not enough glycogen. Protein is required for the building of muscles, which happens after a hard workout. If you burn it up during your workout it can be hard to gain muscle.

Consequently, you want to make sure that when you work out on an empty stomach you don'☐t push yourself too hard- you don't want to pass out. Consider a short run in the morning before your first meal. It'll get you moving and if you keep it light it shouldn't have negative effects.

While it may be hard to exercise during the first few days or weeks, in time, you will get used to fasting, and then you can bring some exercise into your day. However, take care not to exercise excessively on very little food, as it will only bring negative effects.

Chapter Summary

In this chapter we discussed:

- Nutrition during the eating period of intermittent fasting
- Exercise and intermittent fasting

In the next chapter, you will learn more about the benefits of intermittent fasting.

Chapter Three: Benefits of Intermittent Fasting

Why Intermittent Fasting is Beneficial for You

Intermittent fasting is very beneficial in many ways; it offers a lot in terms of good health and the overall well-being of a person. This chapter will discuss some of the ways intermittent fasting is the best thing for your health.

It Aids in Weight-Loss

For many people, this is the number one reason to try intermittent fasting. When you maintain a restricted eating period, you take in fewer calories. This alone will lead to loss of weight. Eating less also encourages your body to tap into the fat reserve it keeps for itself, using it up during the time you are fasting.

The best thing about this for trying to lose weight is that you do not have to keep count of your calorie intake. You will automatically consume fewer calories due to fasting. That is of course unless you make up for the fasting period by binge-eating the rest of the time. So you do still have to watch yourself a little. But if you have the willpower to fast, you certainly have the ability to make sure you eat well when you do eat.

This diet also helps the body to become better at burning fat for the production of energy. Due to the limited time for eating, insulin levels drop thereby permitting the fat cells to release fatty acids. Since the glucose levels are low, the body will be compelled to make use of the fatty acids for energy generation. This energy is used by both the brain and body.

Adherence is very vital to the intermittent fasting diet plan. Several research studies have revealed that quite a large number of people regain their previous weight, or even more, several months after dieting. Why does this happen? The reason is simple; it's because they fail to stick to their diet plans. This is not surprising at all because many diets discourage long-term adherence.

Decreases the risk of Heart Disease

Heart disease has been linked to the lifestyle of a person, with a healthy and regular diet reducing the chances of getting it.

Intermittent fasting has also been seen to reduce the chances of suffering from heart disease. It does this by keeping cholesterol levels in check and improving blood pressure, both of which are risk factors for heart disease.

Reduces the risk of Type 2 Diabetes

Diabetes continues to be a top lifestyle disease among many people all over the world. There is a need to improve how we live to avoid diabetes. Intermittent fasting, therefore, comes as a relief, with its proven ability to reduce the risk of diabetes.

When you fast, you tend to lose weight which then keeps your blood sugar levels down. Your body also becomes more sensitive to insulin, reducing your chances of becoming diabetic. A 2018 study published in the journal, BMJ Case Reports, revealed subjects suffering from Type 2 Diabetes on the intermittent fasting diet reduced body weight and improved post-meal glucose variability. Three of the subjects were able to get off their insulin as well as other oral medication. The lead investigator was Dr. Jason Fung, a kidney expert at the Scarborough and Rouge Hospital in Toronto, Canada.

Improves Brain Function

Intermittent fasting has been seen to improve the function of your brain. Studies suggest that it may improve your memory while preventing short-term memory loss. Professors at the Buck Institute for Research on Aging observed fruit fly larvae that were denied nutrients. They discovered that their brains responded to a scarcity of nutrients the same way ours do during fasting by reducing synaptic functions. This is a way by which the brain conserves energy. When your brain conserves energy it becomes more effective, this is how it stays sharp. It also boosts your cognitive function. It's been shown that fasting also causes an increase in BDNF, a protein in the brain cells. This protein is responsible for learning, cognitive function, and memory.

Intermittent fasting also triggers ketogenesis where the body converts fat into energy and metabolizes fat to ketones. The ketones then feed the brain and improve mental acuity, productivity, and energy. When coupled with the right diet, intermittent fasting also inhibits blood sugar surges caused by high carb diets, which lead to brain fog and mood problems.

Early research also says that this type of fasting may reduce the risk of Alzheimer□'s disease, although this has only been tested on rats.

Prevents Cancer

Intermittent fasting with its positive effects on metabolism has been linked to prevention of cancer. It has also been seen to reduce the effects of cancer when combined with chemotherapy. All this may be due to:

- reduced production of blood glucose

- increased production of cancer-killing cells

- triggered stem cells to regenerate the immune system

- balanced nutritional intake

Slows Down the Aging Process

Would you like to be young forever?

Well, that's impossible, however, you can slow down the aging process and maintain your youth for a while longer. Similar to low-calorie diets, intermittent fasting has been seen to reduce the rate of aging.

Fasting makes your body be able to detoxify and prevent diseases related to old age, which increases your lifespan and makes you age slower. Fasting helps trigger autophagy, a process where our bodies get rid of dead or substandard cells and regenerate damaged proteins.

Intermittent Fasting; The difference between men and women

Intermittent fasting has its benefits. However, it would be good to note that it affects men and women differently. Some women who tried this type of fast have reported having side effects such as:

- No menstrual periods

- Early onset menopause from women as young as 20 years

- Need to eat excessively

- Metabolic disruption

Female Hormones

The effects mentioned are quite serious, especially when you were only trying to lose a few pounds. So why does this happen among women?

The effects can be attributed to the hormonal imbalance caused by fasting. What a woman eats as well as her frequency in eating tends to affect her hormonal balance. A woman's body requires energy to keep hormones at a safe level.

When one has less energy than is required by the body, it tends to dip into energy stored by fat and muscle. Less energy can be caused by eating too little food and not eating for long amounts of time. Using too much stored energy could lead to serious consequences.

Eating less protein for women can lead to a lower count of amino acids which are needed for menstruation to take place. Amino acids tend to lead to the production of growth factors that trigger the thickening of the uterine wall, a process that is necessary for the reproductive cycle. This may be what leads to a lack of menstruation in women on this diet.

Stress and Fasting

The mental state of a woman also tends to affect how fasting affects her. When a woman is under a lot of stress, her hormone levels may change. This is because the body may interpret the stress as a threat to the body, thereby inhibiting production of estrogen. This may stop the reproductive cycle.

Women who are too lean may suffer from infertility due to the lowered production of estrogen in the body. This is because the body may interpret the lack of energy as a threat to fertility, stopping the reproduction cycle.

Furthermore, fasting while you are stressed out may actually be counterproductive. It will further reduce your energy levels adding to the effect of stress on your hormones, thus creating even more problems for you.

Note that not enough estrogen may also make one feel hungry more often than normal. This happens because the metabolism is regulated by estrogen. As such without enough estrogen, the rate of your body's metabolism may increase.

Of course, you can find other ways to lose weight and maintain good health apart from or in addition to fasting. Practice eating whole foods in place of processed foods and exercise regularly.

Men and Fasting

Men are luckier than women, as they tend to benefit from fasting. They generally do not have side effects from fasting. Certainly, they face nothing so serious as potential infertility. Although, men should still be conscious of what they are eating and what they are doing during their fast period. You shouldn't plan to do any intense workout or even operate heavy machinery if you are going through a long fast period.

If you take up intermittent fasting, try to go slow at first; do not spend more than ten hours fasting, and if you notice any of the side effects, it may be better to try other ways to achieve your goals like regular exercise and better nutrition.

Therapeutic Benefits of Intermittent Fasting

- Physical

In addition to its positive effects on the management of diabetes, intermittent fasting has also been proven to reduce seizures, seizure-related brain damage, and even help heal rheumatoid arthritis. Furthermore, there are some positive effects of alternate day fasting on the effects of chemotherapy as well as reducing morbidity that comes with cancer.

- Psychological

Fasting helps us by boosting our willpower through testing our self-control and discipline. During fasting, you consciously make a decision to stay hungry. This means that you have control over your wants and over your body. If you can control your eating habits, you can nurture the willpower to control other aspects of your life as well. Willpower impacts your self-esteem by being able to show self-discipline and control.

Self-control is one of the major indicators of success and happiness.

Intermittent Fasting for Improved Physical Health

- Better metabolism

Intermittent fasting trains your mind and digestive system to consume whatever your body requires for the day within a short window. This encourages a healthy and proportional consumption of food. When you get used to fasting, you learn to eat only when hungry as opposed to pre-conditioned mealtimes.

When done in the correct manner, fasting improves metabolism and as a result, your body will be able to utilize glucose or fats to produce energy.

- Improved wind and endurance

Most athletes build and maintain wind through running as well as doing cardio workouts. In the fitness lingo, VO2 max refers to the maximum quantity of oxygen per sixty seconds, per kg of body weight that one uses during intense exercise. The higher the amount of oxygen you can use at a time, the more output you can do during a workout. The VO2 max is a measure of fitness.

Seasoned athletes have twice the VO2 capacity of untrained people. In a research study conducted by the Department of Exercise Science at George Washington University, in March 2018, the VO2 max levels of a fasted group and a fed group were tested. Both groups started with initial levels of about 3.5L/m. The test group underwent endurance training and changes were evident. The group that fasted registered increased VO2 max as compared to those who didn't.

Intermittent fasting and working out

A majority of people feel better when they train while on the intermittent fasting diet plan. Most of them experienced less hunger throughout the day even though they were eating bigger rations at one time.

Taking in more protein at a single sitting does not make up for low intake at different times of the day. Adjust your fast to have an evenly distributed protein intake throughout the day. BCAAs, branched chain amino acids, shield you from muscle damage, quicken recovery and reduces the breakdown of protein- preventing the feeling of depletion when training in a fasted state.

Please note that taking BCAAs means you are consuming proteins and that's not fasting. However, during training, it's different because they act as a strong source of energy for the muscles. The benefits are greater than breaking your fast.

It's important to know that your method of fasting needs to be in sync with your training's physical demands. The major types of intermittent fasting are tailored to assist individuals, athletes, and bodybuilders maintain good health and boost their performance.

You can also take creatine supplements to increase your lean body mass, muscle fiber, and strength. It is better to take creatine after your training because it will help continue to build muscle when you have finished exercise.

Chapter Summary

In this chapter we learned about:

- The benefits of intermittent fasting

- The drawbacks of IF especially in women

- How to supplement your IF diet when working out

In the next chapter, you will learn about the different types of intermittent fasting plans.

Chapter Four: Intermittent Fasting Plans

The Types of Intermittent Fasting

When you decide to try intermittent fasting, you can choose one of several types of fasting. Each is slightly different from the other, mainly in the frequency and time of eating. If you'□re wondering which type of intermittent fasting regime to try out, read on to learn about each one to know which one will best suit you

Feeding within a restricted time frame: The 16/8 Method

Popularly known as the 16/8 method, this is where you divide the day into a period when you can eat, and a period when you can not eat. It is also known as the daily window fasting. In a day, you would have 8 hours where you can eat anything, after that period you fast for the next 16 hours.

For instance, you can have your first meal at 10 a.m. and eat the last meal of the day at 6 p.m. After that, the next meal you eat would be the next day at 10 a.m. You, therefore, go for 16 hours without taking a meal. This is the most common method but, don't forget, you can choose more hours, even going as far as 20 hours a day, if you wish.

The 16/8 method would go well for someone who likes routine and is not looking to keep track of everything they eat.

- Pros

You can eat anything you feel like within the eight hour window period.

- Cons

The strict nutrition plan can be difficult to adhere to.

Full-day Fasting: the 5/2 Method

In the 5/2 method, every week, you would have 5 days to eat normally, and then pick two non-consecutive days to fast. On the days of your fast, you restrict yourself to a smaller calorie intake - about 200-300 calories.

If you choose Tuesday and Thursday, you can eat what you normally eat on all days except these two and only eat the 200-300 calories and drink water. Full-day fasting tends to increase metabolic rate and also aids in the burning of fat.

- Pros

It is flexible

- Cons

Going a full day without calories can be very difficult and take a lot of willpower

Alternate-day Fasting

You can also take the more intense option of fasting every alternating day. This means you would be eating today and fasting the next day, eating the following day and fasting on the day after that, and so on.

Depending on what you feel will work for you, you don't have to do a total fast, which is when you would go without any food at all. Instead, on the days of your "fast", you can have a diet of a specific number of calories, like 500 calories, and then eat normally on the days you are not fasting. This can be quite uncomfortable and harder to get used to as you will have to go hungry one day while eating comfortably the next.

- Pros

Focuses solely on weight loss. This one cuts the most calories from your week so you will lose weight. Eating less is also said to clear the mind and have detoxifying benefits.

- Cons

It may be easy to follow but you are also more likely to binge eat on your free days.

Skipping meals

The title speaks for itself and this is a much shorter term version of intermittent fasting. The spontaneous person can decide to keep breakfast on one day, then at a later date, skip lunch. This can be planned or natural at times such as when you are busy and lunch period skips your mind, or you are just not hungry.

The Warrior Diet

Here, one eats small amounts of fruit and vegetables all throughout the day and then has one large meal at night. So, you are basically restricting your calories all throughout the day, and feasting at night.

- Pros

The fasting period allows you to snack, so you are not truly going without food.

- Cons

The guidelines on what to eat may be difficult to stick to in the long-term. The strict schedule and meal plan may also interfere with social events.

Each of these methods has its benefits and downside, and one may be easier for you than the other. Find one that will match your schedule and your preferences and stick to it. Remember that each one is unique and a fasting regime which works for one person will not necessarily be the right one for the next person.

Water Fasting

This is the toughest kind of fasting and should never be practiced without supervision from an expert. Some people also regard this as the only real fast. For a span of a few days, you are not allowed to eat or drink anything apart from water. No calories. What this means is that you will be deficient in minerals and vitamins. The main aim of water fasting is usually to detoxify the body and get rid of fat.

If you are coming from an absolutely non-fat adapted state, ketosis kicks in on the second or third day of a water fast, this is when your body resorts to burning fat for energy. Obese people with excess fats may feel a sense of energy during the water fast. Lean people, however, will feel sluggish faster because lean bodies try to preserve energy at all costs.

You need to be warned that since you completely lack food, water fasting is quite uncomfortable. You should start with other fasting patterns before going full throttle on this.

You could also try one of the variations on water fasting which include broth and juice fasting.

Broth fasting involves consumption of bone broth mixed with fats which offer small amounts of protein, electrolytes, and nutrients. Juice contains some of the vitamins and minerals that water lacks. So your calorie count will still basically be at zero, but you will be getting a very slight amount of nutrition as compared to pure water fasting.

Fat Fasting

This type of fast is also known as fast mimicking because it mimics a fast, especially the effects of water fasting. However, you consume healthy fats when fasting, hence the name, fat fasting. Our bodies lack the ability to differentiate dietary fat from metabolizing dietary fat and therefore remains in a state of fasting. This offers you the gains of fasting while enabling you to get the nutrients your body requires to get into ketosis.

Which Intermittent Fasting Plan Should I Choose?

This a commonly asked question. What you choose depends on your goals as well as your fat adapted state. The keto diet assists with fasting since it helps the body to be efficient in converting stored fat into energy. The most obvious goal is always to break through a weight loss plateau. However, some plans are more suited to certain people based on lifestyle. You may need one of the plans with a higher calorie intake because you are on medication that requires food, or because you exercise regularly and doing so on no food at all would be dangerous. There are so many factors so you need to be clear that you are picking what is healthiest for you, you know what your needs are as well as your goals.

The overall benefits of fasting

- Improvement and replenishing of the immune system

- Purging of cancerous cells

- Activation of autophagy

- Reduction of fat tissue via ketosis

- Reduction of C-Reactive protein and oxidative stress

- Improved gene expression that boosts longevity

- Increased BDNF which aids in the survival and growth of new brain neurons as well as improved mental performance

- Improved fasting glucose and healthy stem cell levels

Chapter Summary

We discussed:

- The different types of intermittent fasting plans

- The pros and cons of each plan

In the next chapter, you will learn how to make intermittent fasting work for you.

If you're enjoying this book so far, I would appreciate it so much if you went to Amazon and left a short review.

Chapter Five: Tips to Make Intermittent Fasting Work For You

How to Get Started with Intermittent Fasting

Starting out on intermittent fasting is probably the scariest part for most people because of the uncertainty. There you are having heard all the good things about this type of fasting. You really want to start, and you have no idea how to. Then there is the thought of the hunger pangs you will face.

Missing breakfast? How will you survive? How do you make sure not to mess it up?

It is not nearly as hard as it sounds. All you will need is dedication, and to be able to take it one day at a time. Before you know it, you will have gotten used to it.

Here are a few simple steps to follow to get you started on intermittent fasting:

Have a Clear Purpose

Before you begin to fast, it would be good to have a clearly defined goal. Why are you fasting? Is it because you would like to lose weight? Maybe your family has a history of a medical condition like diabetes and you want to reduce your chances of developing it.

Whatever it is, having a clear goal with defined milestones will help you remain dedicated to the fasting program. When times are tough and you just want to have a snack before your fasting window is over, you will remind yourself of the purpose of your fast and it should keep you going.

To remind yourself of what you want to achieve you can write out your goal on paper and stick it openly on a wall or fridge so that you can see it daily. Even add a reminder on your smartphone so that you don't forget what you're supposed to be doing or what you're doing it for.

Break it Down into Smaller Bits

Sometimes the thought of not eating for more than 10 hours straight can look intimidating.

You picture the agonizing hours and imagine how on a normal day when it□'s almost lunchtime and your day seems to be dragging, you can□'t wait to go eat. But, you can make it less intimidating by breaking it down into hours.

Let us go through a few examples of breaking your fast into manageable bits:

Day one:

- Start by eating what you normally eat. No need to change anything; have breakfast at the normal time - that cup of coffee or tea at your favorite café.
- Eat lunch just as you would any other day, as well as your dinner. When you have your dinner at around 6:30 or 7 p.m., make it your last meal of the day.

- Do not eat anything else for the rest of the night. It is not as hard as it sounds; if you listen to your body, you will realize that most of the time you eat not because you are hungry but just because you feel the need to nibble on something.
- To make it easier, you can find something else to do to keep your mind off the contents of your fridge. Maybe listen to some music, read a book or finish off a project you had started, for instance, the painting you have been putting aside.
- Brush your teeth to make it final that you will eat nothing else for the day. Time will go by and before you know it, it□ is already time to sleep.

Day two

If you make it to the morning, congratulations! You have made it through the first day successfully. Now, the second day is tough, you will need to push your eating time to at least 10 a.m., assuming you are on the 16/8 plan. Take it one hour at a time.

Skipping breakfast is not a foreign thing for most people. You must have done it once or twice before; that time you were running late and only sipped your coffee before you rushed to the office, or when you slept in and woke up past 12 p.m. and had lunch for your first meal.

Think of this particular fasting period like any of these past instances. Go on with your normal routine; get some work done, maybe update your planner or attend meetings as planned.

At 10 a.m. or later, you can have your first meal of the day. Go on with your day, have lunch, maybe a little bit later as you might not be hungry at 1 p.m. and then have dinner at 7 p.m.

What if you slip up?

You may have gotten overwhelmed somewhere in between, sneaked in a snack in the middle of the night, or ate a doughnut in the morning. If this happens, don☐'t be so hard on yourself. Just continue with your fast and try again the next day.

Tips for intermittent fasting
1. Choose the fasting type that best suits you

Research on all the types of fasting and find one that will go well with your personality, routine, and your lifestyle.

2. Drink lots of water

While on your fast, no matter what kind you choose, you can and should drink water. Take advantage of this by drinking as much water as you can. It helps keep the hunger pangs at bay while you are on the fasting period.

3. Keep your time occupied

A good side effect of fasting is becoming more productive. You don'☐t want periods of time where you have nothing to distract you from the need to eat something. Boredom makes you want to eat and so does idleness. Keep yourself busy all throughout the day.

4. Eat healthily

During your eating window, you want to make sure that you are having a balanced diet. Eating healthy foods is especially important for best results if you are fasting to lose weight. As we covered earlier, this includes some protein, healthy fats and lots of fruits.

5. It gets easier

You won'☐t always have to work so hard to make it through hours without food. With time, you will get used to it, and it will come to you effortlessly.

6. Avoid or reschedule intense workouts

Intense workouts will make you ravenous and unable to concentrate on anything else. Try to avoid them, especially when you are just starting out on intermittent fasting. You can resume exercise at a convenient time, preferably within your eating window later on.

How to stay motivated with intermittent fasting

Fasting may be hard to keep up with over time, especially if it is simply a monotonous routine. So, how do you keep at it, stay motivated, and reap the benefits?

1. Remind yourself that your body can survive a little hunger

The biggest issue when it comes to intermittent fasting is the part where you actually have to stay without eating for long periods of time. This is where most people fail, slipping up and eating something when they shouldn'☐t. Yet think about it, most of the time we eat not because we are hungry really, but due to boredom, stress or anxiety.

Feeling the urge to eat something doesn'☐t always mean you are hungry. You probably feel like sleeping while at work at times too, but you wouldn't, and probably don't really need to.

So, when you realize that your body can not only survive but actually thrive on far less calories than you would normally consume, you can take the hunger, and your body will thank you for it.

2. Drink lots of fluids

You can have water, tea, even coffee, both during your eating window and when you are in the fasting period. When you start to feel hungry, gulp down some water or herbal tea.

These drinks will help you get through the hard days. Coffee serves to make you feel good and actually works as a hunger suppressant so it will help keep you going during your fast.

3. Mix up your meals

You can make very interesting meals if you put some effort into it. Find different ingredients with a wide range of nutrients. Remember what we discussed earlier about making sure you have different food groups; protein, carbs, and veggies. Keeping it fun and different will motivate you to go ahead with your intermittent fasting, looking forward to trying new flavors and textures.

4. Treat yourself to something special every once in a while

While you can□'t have chocolate and large, meaty burgers every day, you can always treat yourself to one after a while. It can be your own pat on the back after a successful fasting period- perhaps you've been going strong for 2 or 3 weeks.

This can be something other than food. Fasting can help you save your money since you won't be eating out as often as you used to. Thank yourself for the effort and indulge in a shopping spree, buy yourself a beautiful outfit, or that cool gadget you've had your eye on for a while. You deserve it.

Common mistakes

There are several common mistakes in intermittent fasting that you would do well to avoid:

1. Eating the wrong food

While you are not restricted in what you eat when practicing intermittent fasting, the kind of food you eat matters a lot. You can't eat only junk foods while fasting and expect to lose weight.

Your body needs the right foods to provide the right nutrients to build it up, and junk food won't cut it. Look at the foods we discussed in Chapter 2 to get the best foods to eat while fasting.

Also, avoid overeating or undereating during your feeding window. Both of these may lead to negative results, including a weak body and no weight loss.

2. Choosing a plan which you can't keep up with

We looked at different types of intermittent fasting plans earlier and saw that there are several of them, each a bit different from the next.

You may choose one that you can't keep up with, for whatever reason, and give up on fasting after a short while. Take your time looking at each and choose one that will suit you best to increase your chances of succeeding.

3. Giving up

I will admit that the first few days are quite hard. One common mistake people make is deciding to give up very early in their fasting period. A few days or a week won't cut it. You can't see the benefits of a method unless you give it time to actually work, so do persevere for a while longer before deciding to quit.

4. Pushing yourself too hard

Sometimes one may push themselves, doing too much too soon. For instance, if you have just started fasting, and were eating more than 6 times a day before, you can't just jump into a 20-hour fasting period. Start small and build up. You will need to ease into the hours, starting with fewer hours and building up from there. The same applies to exercise when you begin to fast.

It doesn't sound so hard now, does it? Take the leap and start fasting today with these easy and doable tips. These are but a few useful insights to help you stay on track in the journey of intermittent fasting. Embrace the tips on staying motivated and avoid the common mistakes which could derail you.

Chapter Summary

This chapter discussed:

- How to get started on the intermittent fasting diet plan
- Tips for intermittent fasting
- How to stay motivated
- Common mistakes to avoid on this diet

In the next chapter, you will be introduced to the Ketogenic diet.

Chapter Six: Introduction to the Ketogenic Diet

With all its popularity today, it might surprise you to learn that the ketogenic diet has been used for nearly a century. Because of that, the diet is very well studied and has been shown scientifically to be safe for most people.

History of the Ketogenic Diet

The ketogenic diet was originally developed by Dr. Russell Wilder at the famous Mayo Clinic in Rochester, Minnesota. Back in 1924 when he first invented the diet, Dr. Wilder wasn't looking for a weight loss mechanism but a way to control epileptic seizures in children. The diet proved quite successful, and the only reason it fell out of the public eye was the development of pharmaceutical methods to control epilepsy.

However, in the 1990s Jim Abrahams, a producer in Hollywood, revived the diet to treat his son, who was not responding to conventional anticonvulsant drugs. Lucky for Abrahams' son, he was being treated at Johns Hopkins Hospital in Baltimore, where they were still using the ketogenic diet as an option to control seizures. The ketogenic diet wound up being so successful that Abrahams established a nonprofit group to share the news with other families impacted by epilepsy. There was even a made-for-television movie about the case that starred Meryl Streep called "...First Do No Harm."

The Basic Premise of the Ketogenic Diet

So, what is this magical diet anyway? It's a way to power your body on fat instead of carbohydrates. Rather than eating a broad range of foods from all the different food groups, you eat primarily fat and protein, with very few starchy foods like potatoes, bread, and pasta.

The next chapter will lay out more of the science behind the diet. Meanwhile, let's take a look at some of the basic tenets of the diet, so you can determine whether or not it's for you. After all, a diet is only as good as your ability to stick to it, right?

First, let's dispel the myth that you need to eat a lot of carbohydrates (AKA carbs) to have energy throughout the day. The only part of your body that needs glycogen, which your body makes from carbs, is the brain. Otherwise, fat is a much more efficient source of fuel, and guess what? If you have weight to lose, you already have a built-in storage of fuel!

If the ketogenic diet sounds a lot like other low-carb diets today, you're right - it does. But there are a few key differences. Compared to the Atkins diet and the Paleo diet, the ketogenic diet uses much more regimented portions of each food group to ensure the diet works. In fact, you'll be eating a diet that's about 70 to 90 percent fat. The normal American diet is much higher in carbohydrates and lower in fat.

Calorie Counting on the Ketogenic Diet

You may be wondering if you need to count calories on the ketogenic diet. The answer is maybe. Some people have great success with keto simply changing the ratios of their food groups to a higher percentage of fat and protein. As long as they don't consume a high volume of food and don't get their calories from junk food, they lose weight and feel great.

Other people find they need more structure to their ketogenic diet. Maybe they have a hard time with impulse or binge eating. Perhaps they struggle with portion control (a common problem in the United States). For these people, counting calories and percentages of macronutrients (fat, protein, carbohydrates, etc.) helps them lose weight with keto.

While this book doesn't get into the calorie content of foods allowed on the ketogenic diet, never fear. You can easily find "keto calculators" online, and there are even keto apps for mobile devices. By weighing and measuring everything you eat according to these calculators, you can ensure you are eating the right number of calories for your dietary needs and for your desired weight loss. Once you hit your target weight, you can use the same calculator to count the new caloric intake you need to maintain your weight.

If you start the ketogenic diet using the "eyeball" method - simply eating the foods on the approved list without counting calories - and you don't lose weight within a week or so, you probably want to switch to a keto calculator and make adjustments to your intake. It might mean eating less food in total, or it could mean you need to change the source of your calories.

Dieting is a uniquely personal experience; what works for one person doesn't necessarily work for another. There are lots of factors that can affect how you need to tweak your diet, such as your sex, age, hormonal balance, medical conditions, amount of exercise, stress level, current weight, and weight loss goals. It's okay if you take a week or two at the start to set yourself up for success down the road.

Foods Allowed on the Ketogenic Diet

While you'll learn more specifics in later chapters about what you can and cannot eat on the ketogenic diet, understand that you'll be shaking up the traditional food pyramid as you probably know it. At the bottom of the pyramid are all the foods you are encouraged to eat on a ketogenic diet, like meat, eggs, oils, and non-starchy vegetables. In the middle of the pyramid, you'll find low-carb vegetables, such as cauliflower, broccoli, and tomatoes. The next layer is made up of full-fat dairy products, and at the top you'll find foods you can eat in very limited quantities, like berries and watermelon.

You'll be able to drink as much tea and coffee as you like, and you'll be drinking a lot of water too. Limited amounts of alcohol are allowed based on their sugar content.

Foods You Have to Give Up on the Ketogenic Diet

As you now know, there are some foods you will be abstaining from on the keto diet because they are too high in carbohydrates. These include soda, juice, potatoes, bread, grains, dried beans, and processed foods.

While this may seem punitive, the diet won't work if you eat these foods. Because it is scientifically based on how your body metabolizes different macronutrients, the keto diet must be adhered to in a strict manner. Don't worry, you'll learn lots of ways to adapt your favorite foods and prepare new ones later in this book.

Benefits of the Ketogenic Diet

Lest you start to think this diet is all punishment and little reward, take a look at the benefits of a keto lifestyle. Bookmark this page, so you can refer to it frequently when you first start the diet to remind yourself why you are making this big change to your eating habits.

Numerous conditions, in addition to epilepsy, have responded well to the ketogenic diet, including:

- Insulin resistance, pre-diabetes, and diabetes.
- Chronic pain.
- Mood disorders.
- Digestive disorders.
- Dermatologic conditions.
- High cholesterol and high triglycerides.

Of course, excess weight and obesity respond to it too - you will lose weight. In some limited cases, even cancer patients have improved while on the keto diet.

Insulin Resistance, Pre-Diabetes, and Diabetes

In addition to having been well studied for epilepsy, the ketogenic diet has been researched for other conditions, including problems related to blood sugar, like pre-diabetes and diabetes. In one trial at Duke University, participants who followed the ketogenic diet witnessed a significant drop in their hemoglobin a1c, which is a marker for high blood sugar.

Their blood sugar levels dropped, as did their triglycerides, a component of cholesterol. Many also enjoyed a large weight loss of nearly 20 pounds on average. The Duke study participants were even able to reduce or eliminate their diabetes medications.

Insulin resistance can be a precursor to diabetes and indicate a greater risk of cardiovascular disease. It means your cells aren't as sensitive to the insulin the body makes to break down sugars as they should be. Insulin sensitivity can be restored with a ketogenic diet.

If you have diabetes or are on medications for your blood sugar or cholesterol, you may be able to improve your health with a ketogenic diet. Consult your doctor about making this dietary change, and do not discontinue any medications without your physician's permission. If the diet is successful, you may be able to taper off drugs or insulin slowly, so, once again, make sure you work with a doctor to create a plan that's unique to your needs.

Chronic Pain

Eating a diet that's high in carbohydrates isn't just bad for your blood sugar and weight. Sugar can cause inflammation in your joints, so eliminating it from your diet may improve conditions like arthritis and idiopathic pain-the pain of unknown origin.

Additionally, the same nerve pathways that are involved in seizures are activated when you feel pain. Neuropathic pain, such as that suffered by people with serious diabetes, is a new area of research for the ketogenic diet and may be relieved with the keto food regimen.

Mood Disorders

It is difficult and sometimes impossible for doctors to know the root cause of every mood problem. Some people are believed to be born "hardwired" for mood problems, while others may develop them as the result of their life situation.

Nevertheless, anticonvulsant drugs are often prescribed for mood disorders. Because the ketogenic diet prevents seizures like anticonvulsants, it is thought that it could also have the same effect on mood disorders.

Furthermore, the stabilized blood sugar and the increased energy and mental clarity many people find on the ketogenic diet may also play a role in improving mood. When you add in weight loss and less chronic pain, people whose life circumstances contribute to depression and mood swings may find relief with keto.

Digestive Disorders

There are numerous digestive problems that have been shown to be relieved by following a ketogenic diet. It's natural that a diet without grains would be helpful for celiac disease, in which the body cannot tolerate gluten. However, the ketogenic diet is also beneficial for IBS (irritable bowel syndrome), with a reduction in belly pain and diarrhea that typically accompany this condition.

Have you been told you have a digestive yeast overload or "leaky gut syndrome?" The ketogenic diet eliminates foods that feed yeast (carbohydrates) and lets you stop fueling candida (yeast). When your gut flora returns to normal, you'll see less bloating, and you may even have more energy. Your intestines can heal themselves naturally and prevent the spill of candida into the bloodstream from leaks in the intestinal walls.

Dermatologic Conditions

With your skin being the body's largest organ, it's no surprise it would benefit from the ketogenic diet and the elimination of sugars that cause inflammation and premature signs of aging. Some people have also found relief from acne and rosacea with the ketogenic diet.

High Cholesterol and Triglycerides

When you get your cholesterol taken by a blood test, your triglycerides are measured. High triglycerides can put you at risk of heart attack, blood clots, and stroke. You can also develop liver and pancreas problems from long-term high triglycerides.

Surprisingly, in spite of its high dietary fat content, the ketogenic diet usually results in lower triglycerides for followers. If you have high triglycerides and decide to try the ketogenic diet, let your doctor know, so you can monitor your cholesterol periodically and see if the diet is having the desired effect.

Chapter Summary

This chapter gave you an introduction to the popular ketogenic diet.

- The ketogenic diet has been around for nearly 100 years and is well studied.
- This diet involves eating a high percentage of fat and protein and almost no carbohydrates.
- Many ketogenic dieters find relief from a multitude of health conditions, in addition to losing weight.

In the next chapter, you will learn about the science behind the ketogenic diet.

Chapter Seven: How the Ketogenic Diet Works

In the previous chapter, you learned the basics of the ketogenic diet and that it involves drastically reducing your carbohydrate intake. This chapter will teach you why the diet is structured the way it is and why adhering to the "rules" will boost your success.

The Process of Ketogenesis

You learned in the previous chapter that the ketogenic diet requires you to eat a lot of fat and a good bit of protein, with very few carbohydrates. Why? This fat forms a very efficient fuel, but it's not used directly. First, the body breaks down the fat in the liver, using a process called "ketogenesis," hence the name of the diet.

Ketogenesis produces energy in free fatty acids, which are ideal for your muscles to use in both daily activities and exercise. It also causes the body to form acetoacetate, which is then formed into ketones. Ketones can function as a substitute for glycogen, which you may recall is made from carbohydrates.

Have you heard keto fans talking about being "in ketosis" or "keto-adapted?" That means they have gotten used to being on the ketogenic diet, and their body has adapted to using fats for fuel instead of carbs.

Probably the greatest challenge for ketogenic dieters is the first week - before the body becomes keto-adapted. It generally takes a minimum of three to four days to become used to the diet and for your body to start producing ketones.

How will you know when you have made the shift? You can buy "keto sticks" that check for ketones in your urine. Also, the initial fatigue and fogginess most people experience when they first start the ketogenic diet subsides. Your carb cravings will be less urgent, and you'll start to see less of an up-and-down feeling to your energy levels.

The aim of the ketogenic diet is the improvement of one's well-being through a change in metabolism. Here is what you need to know about the ketogenic diet:

- Who is not allowed to follow this diet
- How to begin this diet plan
- What to be concerned of with low carb diets
- Side effects of this diet
- Benefits of the ketogenic diet

Before starting a ketogenic diet plan, one should consult with a medical practitioner. This is mandatory so that you are informed of any pre-existing health conditions.

Basics

There are several ways by which one can implement a low carb ketogenic diet plan. But the majority of them requires one to follow a higher fat, moderate protein, and low carb food plan. One of the most popular ketogenic diets is the Atkins diet. Several people believe that ketogenic diets are diets high in protein, but this is not true. These disparities revolve around the amount of carbohydrate and protein allowed on a day to day basis:

- A ketogenic diet plan needs one to track the number of carbs in the foods consumed and reduction of carbohydrate intake to an average of 40 grams in a day. For other people, consuming less than 100 grams in a day may be effective. However, this carb level is too high for the majority of people to achieve ketosis. Additionally, the daily requirement for protein should be triggered by the aim or ideal body weight or lean body mass. Intake of protein also depends on height, gender and the amount of exercise that one does. Too much protein consumption can interfere with ketosis. The balance of calories after calculation of carbs and protein needs will be from fats. The ratios make sure that majority of people enter ketosis and remain in that state.
- The nutrient intake on a ketogenic diet works out to about 70-75% of calories from fat, 20-25% from protein and 5-10% from carbohydrates every day when calories are not restricted. Even though counting calories is not needed, it is vital to understand how the macronutrient percentages can be affected by the consumption of calories.

The secret to implementing a ketogenic diet in the correct manner is to keep in mind that you are alternating foods containing carbohydrates with more fats and moderate protein.

Fats have little effect, if any, on your levels of blood sugar as well as insulin. Protein affects both the levels of blood sugar and insulin. If you consume a lot of protein for your ideal body weight, it can increase your levels of blood sugar and insulin will also be increased by protein temporarily. Higher levels will affect the production of ketone bodies. Moreover, having a diet that has a lot of lean protein (with less fat) could make you sick.

How to Start a Ketogenic Diet Plan

One should understand the consequences of what will take place when intake of carbohydrate drops. You could follow the tips below:

- Get a carb counter guide
This will assist you in learning and recalling the number of carbs in the foods that you eat. Counting of carbs is important in this diet plan and it is important for one to understand how it is done.

- Go on a carbohydrate sweep
Inspect your food area and get rid of all foods that are high in carbs. This includes even whole grains.

- Restock the kitchen

Do this so that the foods that are low in carbohydrates are available. This will aid in keeping you on the right path.

- This diet is not a diet that needs special foods. You don't need to buy low carb packaged foodstuffs. Ketogenic foods are not highly processed foods. They are real whole foods that are close to their natural state. The only exception is the category of artificial sweeteners which are highly processed.
- Be ready to spend more time in the kitchen. This diet is all about cooking and eating foods that are real. If you don't know how to cook, learn now.
- Give your meals thought and plan them. This will aid you in buying the right foods from the grocery store.
- Replace old habits with new ones.
- Stay hydrated. As you lower carbohydrate intake, the kidneys will begin dumping excess water. Ensure that you take a lot of water to replace what is lost. If you find yourself experiencing headaches and muscle cramps, it means that you need more water.
- Steer clear of high carb foods because they will increase your levels of sugar and insulin. Additionally, cereal grains like wheat are toxic for most people.
- Consider taking natural supplements.
- You can also buy some testing kits so that you can find out if you are in ketosis. The reagent strip should not register as deep purple if you are using ketones as a fuel source.

- Keep a spreadsheet to track daily food intake and carb counts. Use one of the online food intake trackers or write it down in a journal. In addition to keeping you on track, it will also aid you in recording the type of foods that you eat, how you feel, and the changes that you make.
- Think of any social distractions and find ways of handling them.
- You should also avoid focusing on your weight. Stop checking your weight on a daily basis. The body's weight varies on a daily basis because of differences in water intake and absorption. You will not have the ability to track fat loss every day. You can check your weight once every seven days.
- Lastly, learn how to stop craving sugar.

Chapter Summary

This chapter discussed:

- The process of Ketogenesis
- The basics of the Ketogenic diet
- Getting started on the Ketogenic diet

In the next chapter, you will learn the advantages as well as the risks of the Ketogenic diet.

Chapter Eight: Pros and Cons of The Ketogenic Diet

Is the Ketogenic Diet Safe?

The dangers of low-carb diets are mostly just myths - people who have a limited understanding of how these diets work come up with them. Their main fears are related to fat intake and the ketosis process.

Fears Regarding Fat

A majority of people are troubled by this diet plan because they are afraid of increasing the amount of fat that they consume. This is true, you will increase fat intake, especially saturated fats. For decades, people have been told how bad fat is. This message has been repeated over and over again, but it's not always true.

A diet high in carbs raises blood sugar levels as well as insulin. All that sugar and insulin is inflammatory. Even though saturated fat is healthy, it was blamed for causing heart ailments because it was studied when eaten in conjunction with high carb diets. A ketogenic diet that is high in saturated fats and very low in carbohydrate will reduce inflammation.

Saturated Fats in the Low-Carb Diet Context

According to research produced by John Hopkins medical school, saturated fat has no harm in the context of a low-carb diet. The ketogenic diet is healthier because the increased consumption of the saturated fat increases one's HDL cholesterol while at the same time, a diet low in carbs reduces the levels of triglycerides. These two factors are important when it comes to heart ailments.

The closer the triglyceride/HDL ratio is to 1, the healthier the heart. Heart disease is caused by a high intake of carbohydrates rather than a high consumption of saturated fat and cholesterol. The best way to monitor these levels is to have a full blood test before you begin the ketogenic diet then follow the diet plan for ninety days. After that, do another blood test.

General Side Effects of the Ketogenic Diet

At first, switching to a ketogenic diet plan may be difficult because the metabolism of one's body is adapting to fat burning rather than depending on glucose. However, it's good to know that most of the symptoms can be avoided. During the first seven days on this diet, your blood sugar will drop and you may experience an overload of insulin and reactive hypothermia. This usually happens to people who are resistant to insulin.

It takes approximately three days to burn through all the glycogen that is stored in the muscles and liver. A ketogenic diet also has the ability to alter the water and mineral balance of a person's body, so, adding extra salt to food and taking mineral supplements may be helpful. Try taking sodium, potassium, and magnesium on a daily basis to reduce the side effects. These supplements are easily found online or your local drug store.

Benefits and Dangers

If you follow a ketogenic diet plan and adapt to it, you will feel much better and healthier. One of the health gains of this diet is that it will lower your fasting blood sugar as well as levels of insulin. You will feel more energized.

In case you have doubts, please remember that there is a lot of credible research that has shown how following a ketogenic diet plan is not harmful to the health of humans. It is only when one consumes too much fat and a lot of carbs that you negatively impact on your health. The sugar that comes from carbohydrates increases the levels of insulin and those high levels of insulin interrupt your normal metabolism of fat. More fat is then stored or circulated in the bloodstream.

This results in the metabolic syndrome and weight gain that is linked with a resistance to insulin. Then the health issues associated with a diet high in carbohydrates, not a ketogenic diet plan, begin.

- This diet aids in losing weight

A ketogenic diet is an effective way of losing weight while also lowering risks of ailments. Research has revealed that ketogenic diets are far more effective than the usually recommended low-fat diets. Furthermore, the ketogenic diet is so filling that you can shed weight without counting calories or denying yourself good food.

Another study also found out that people on a ketogenic diet lost two times more weight than those on a calorie-restricted low-fat diet plan. Their triglyceride, as well as HDL levels, also improved. It was also found out in a separate study that people on a ketogenic diet lost three times more weight than those on diabetes recommended diet.

Several reasons exist as to why a ketogenic diet is better than a low-fat diet. One of them is the increased consumption of protein which offers benefits. In a nutshell, ketogenic diets aid one in losing weight better than diets with low fat. All this happens without hunger.

- Ketogenic diet for diabetes and prediabetes

This diet enables you to lose excess fat, which is closely connected to type 2 diabetes, prediabetes, as well as metabolic syndrome. Several studies have been done to prove that this diet aids with diabetes. One of them found out that this diet improved the sensitivity of your body to insulin by a whopping 75%.

Another also investigated people with type 2 diabetes. It found out that seven out of the twenty-one participants were able to stop all medications related to diabetes. This diet has the ability to boost insulin sensitivity and trigger loss of fat, which results in the improvement of type 2 diabetes and prediabetes.

Other Health Benefits

The ketogenic diet originally came about as a tool for the treatment of neurological disorders like epilepsy. It also has the ability to improve body fat, HDL levels, blood pressure, and blood sugar. Furthermore, this diet is also being used in the treatment of several cancer types and slowing of tumor growths. It also reduces the symptoms of Alzheimer's and slows down its progress.

In epilepsy, it reduces seizures.

It improves the symptoms of Parkinson's.

Since this diet reduces the levels of insulin, it plays a key role in polycystic ovary syndrome.

A study also found out that the ketogenic diet reduces concussions and aids in recovery for those with brain injuries.

For those suffering from acne, lower levels of insulin, as well as consumption of less sugar and processed foods is beneficial. Here is a breakdown of some more of the benefits from the carb reduction in a ketogenic diet.

- It suppresses appetite in a good way

Feeling hungry is the worst side effect of being on a diet. It is one of the major reasons that many people give up on their dieting programs. One of the advantages of a low carb diet is that it leads to an automatic appetite reduction. Studies have shown that when people cut carbs and consume more protein and fat, they end up consuming fewer calories.

- A lot of fat loss happens in the abdominal cavity

Not all fats in the body are alike. Where fat is stored determines how it affects health as well as the risk of illness. It is important to know that we have fat under the skin and in the abdominal cavity. The fat that tends to be around the organs is what is known as visceral fat. A lot of fat in such areas can trigger inflammation, resistance to insulin, and is responsible for metabolism syndrome. Diets low in carbs are quite effective in the reduction of such abdominal fat.

- Reduction of triglycerides

Triglycerides are molecules of fat. Consumption of carbs drives up levels of triglycerides, especially sugar. When a person cuts down on carbs, they experience a reduction in blood triglycerides.

- Increased levels of good cholesterol

The higher the levels of HDL, the lower the risk of heart ailments. One of the best ways to raise levels of HDL is to consume fat and diets low in carbs.

- Reduction of blood sugar and insulin levels

When we consume carbohydrates, they are broken down into glucose in the digestive tract. Afterward, they enter the bloodstream and raise the levels of blood sugar. Since high levels of blood sugar are toxic, the body responds with insulin. For healthy people, the rapid response of insulin minimizes the blood sugar surge in order to prevent it from being harmful to us.

However, many people have a resistance to insulin. This means that the body does not detect its own insulin making it difficult for the body to absorb blood sugar into the cells. This can lead to type 2 diabetes. By reducing your intake of carbs, you eliminate the need for insulin, and won't build up a resistance.

- Reduction of blood pressure

Low carb diets are effective in the reduction of blood pressure which further reduces the risk of diseases.

- The ketogenic diet is the most effective in the treatment of metabolic syndrome

The symptoms are:

- Abdominal obesity
- Increased blood pressure
- Increased fasting blood sugar levels
- High triglycerides
- Low HDL levels

All these symptoms improve on a low carb diet.

- The ketogenic diet improves the pattern of LDL cholesterol

This is bad cholesterol and is linked to risk for heart attacks. A diet that is low on carbs transforms LDL particles from small to large, and at the same time reduces the number of LDL particles that float into the bloodstream.

Ketones

These are chemical structures of three ketone bodies: acetone, acetoacetic acid, and beta-hydroxybutyric acid. They are produced by the liver from fatty acids when we have low food intake or when we fast completely. They are also produced when we have low carb intake, starve, or we intensely exercise.

The ketones are then picked up and converted to enter the citric acid cycle. From there, they are oxidized to release energy. Ketone bodies are produced through intense gluconeogenesis. This is the process of producing glucose from non-carb sources but does not include fatty acids. Therefore, they are produced by the liver together with newly produced glucose after the liver's reserves have run out. They run out just within 24 hours when fasting.

Also, ketone bodies have a unique scent which can be detected in the breath of people in ketosis and ketoacidosis. The scent is similar to nail polish remover. The ketone bodies are channeled into the bloodstream from the liver. The ketone bodies are then taken from the blood and converted into energy. The availability of high levels of ketone bodies in the bloodstream during starvation or during long periods of exercise and type 1 diabetes is called ketosis. In its extreme state, it is referred to as ketoacidosis.

Ketone bodies cannot be utilized by the liver for energy because they lack the responsible enzymes. In normal people, ketone bodies are constantly produced by the liver and the concentration is maintained at around 1 mg/dl. Their removal through urine is quite low and cannot be detected by using normal urine exams.

When the rate of production of ketone bodies is more than their usage, their concentration increases in the bloodstream. This is referred to as ketonemia. This is succeeded by ketonuria, which is the removal of ketone bodies through urine. Ketonemia and ketonuria is referred to as ketosis. People who take diets that are low in carbs develop ketosis. This is at times referred to as nutritional ketosis.

A blood test that is done in a laboratory is the most accurate and sure way of measuring ketones. It is recommended for people that suffer from diabetes whenever they feel ill. Symptoms such as nausea, vomiting, or pain in the abdomen normally occur when the blood sugar is high. This may mean that you are suffering from diabetic ketoacidosis.

Home tests for ketones done on the blood or urine:

- Monitors a person suffering from diabetes

- Monitors a person on a diet with low carbs or high fat consumption

- Monitors a person who has difficulty eating

How the test is done in a laboratory

- A band that is elastic will be wrapped around the upper arm to stop blood flow. This enlarges the veins below the band and makes it easier to needle the vein.

- The pierced area is cleaned using alcohol

- The needle is inserted in the vein and more than one needle stick may be required

- A tube is then attached to the needle so that it is filled with blood.

- The band is then removed from the arm when enough blood is collected.

- A gauze pad or cotton ball is applied over the pierced point as the needle is removed

- Pressure is then applied to the site and bandaged

Blood tests at home

Some blood sugar meters can be used in measuring blood ketones. You use the same method you use for measuring blood sugar.

If your blood sugar is at a normal range, and you are experiencing weight loss, the presence of ketones may be perfectly normal. However, if you are diabetic, you need to watch your ketones and blood sugar. You should test for ketones if:

- Your blood sugar is over 300
- Your skin is flushed or changes color
- You vomit, have nausea or pains in the abdomen

- You feel lethargic
- You are thirstier than usual
- You have problems breathing
- Your breath smells fruity

Losing weight by achieving optimal ketosis

The first and most important thing is to select a diet that is low in carbs.

This is not recommended for sufferers of type 1 diabetes. The trick is to eat more fat. More fat in food fills you more. This will make sure that you don't eat a lot of protein and carbohydrates. The insulin levels will go down and enable you to reach optimal ketosis.

Being in optimal ketosis for a longer period of time will ensure that one experiences a maximum hormonal effect from eating a low carb diet. You can also order a ketone meter online and measure.

Ketosis, disease treatment, and health

In addition to burning fat, ketosis is beneficial for overall health and treatment of disease. Several cancers feed on glucose. Studies show that cancer has no ability to utilize ketones for the production of fuel, therefore they starve. Normal body cells have the metabolic flexibility to use ketone bodies for fuel. On the contrary, cancer does not.

Ketosis and improved focus and brain function

One of the causes of neurotoxicity is too much glucose. So, if the glucose supply is reduced, and the brain is prompted to burn ketones for fuel, you can reduce negative brain effects. Ketogenic diets also improve the function of the brain through the process of clean fuel production.

Ketosis satiety

Your body *should be* in ketosis. The body should be able to utilize both ketones and glucose to produce fuel. As a sugar burner, the body has only one source to select from, and that is glucose. As a fat burner, it has two sources to select from. Another benefit of fat burning is that it provides energy that is steady as well as long term. Also, when the body does not need sugar constantly, one achieves satiation and a reduced feeling of hunger.

Ketosis and mental performance

Let us first look at how Ketosis is linked to energy. The basis of the Keto diet is that is that it makes use of a specially tailored balance of macronutrients to get a specific response from one's body. When on a Ketogenic diet, you eat normal amounts of protein, higher amounts of fats with low carbs- less than 50 grams in a day. When you take small amounts of carbs, the body will respond as it does during starvation. Rather than utilizing the primary source of energy (glucose), the brain pulls from its alternative energy source, fat.

It is good to point out that before fats are used by our bodies, first the liver has to convert them to Ketone bodies. After, these Ketone bodies are used as energy for the body and brain in the absence of glucose. This is Ketosis. Since you now have a basic understanding of how Ketosis works, let us now talk about how it can be used to improve your productivity as well as your mental state.

Ketones improve your brain's function

The standard diet of western countries is deficient in many aspects including fatty acids. This is not good for our health since we need them for the proper functioning of the body and brain. As we've discussed, It is a well-known fact that Ketones benefits people with neurodegenerative illnesses such as epilepsy, Alzheimer's, Parkinson's and aging-related cognitive diseases. Ketone bodies can be helpful because affected brains are unable to utilize enough of the available glucose to handle perception and cognition. A Keto diet helps by offering an alternative source of energy.

Increased intake of fat from Keto diets has been shown to improve brain function in ways such as:

- A study published by the American diabetes association revealed that type 1 diabetics showed improved cognitive performance and preserved brain function during hypoglycemia after taking medium chain triglycerides derived from coconut oil (Keto diets also increase triglycerides)

- Those with Alzheimer's have seen improved memory scores that may be linked to the amount of Ketones levels present.
- Ketones from a very low-carb diet have also been shown to improve mild cognitive impairment in seniors.

You may be asking yourself if a Keto diet brings a true cognitive improvement for healthy people. Does Ketosis encourage better health in the brains of average people? One thing is for sure; the Keto diet benefits the brain because of its neuroprotective properties. With this in mind, we need to consider essential fatty acids (omega 3 and omega 6) which are vital for proper brain health and function.

Most of our brain tissue consists of fatty acids even though our bodies can't make them on their own. Therefore, we must get the fatty acids from a healthy Ketogenic diet. When we are in a Ketogenic state, Ketones are used by the brain to generate adenosine triphosphate, a molecule that is used for carrying energy where it is required for metabolism within the cells. Even though glucose is the primary source of energy for our bodies, Ketones are actually a more efficient source of energy and they have the power to reduce the amount of destructive free radicals we produce. Within the brain, energy is very important because it protects it from oxidative stress which negatively affects one's mental performance and brain aging.

Ketosis and focus

A diet that is not well-balanced leads to lack of mental clarity, foggy brain, poor memory and the inability to stay focused on tasks. The two factors involved here are:

- Glutamate- a neurotransmitter that boosts stimulation in the body and is useful for brain functioning and learning.
- Gamma-aminobutyric acid (GABA)- the main neurotransmitter in the body that reduces stimulation.

Any time you talk, think or process information, glutamate is involved; as intelligence increases, glutamate receptors on the cells increase. But just as we know that anything is bad in excess, so is glutamate. Glutamate should be able to convert into GABA but at times, this conversion doesn't happen as it is supposed to. Glutamate is responsible for almost 100% of the brain's synaptic connections and the brain can over-process and will not have GABA available to assist in reduced stimulation.

As a result, if our bodies have excess glutamate and less GABA, we are likely to experience brain fog, troubled concentration, reduced social behavior as well as increased anxiety. Ketones provide the brain with an alternate source of energy and allow it to efficiently process the extra glutamate into GABA. Ketones increase the production of GABA, thereby reducing the number of extra neurons that are firing in the brain and boosts mental focus.

Consequently, you will experience reduced anxiety and stress.

Ketones and memory

Another manner in which Ketone bodies reduce free radicals in your brain is by improving the efficiency and levels of energy in the mitochondria which are responsible for energy production. Ketosis helps in making new mitochondria and increasing ATP in the brain's memory cells.

Please note that within the first few weeks of starting the Keto diet, you may experience some mental fog or headaches because when you reduce carb intake your body uses up the leftover glucose. You don't need to worry though because this is temporary and is due to the body flushing out electrolytes from the diuretic effect of Ketosis. To counter these side effects until your body has adapted, drink more water.

Low carb diets have a wonderful way of providing the brain with energy through a process called Ketogenesis and gluconeogenesis. Ketones are produced in small quantities when you go for several hours without eating such as after a full night's sleep. However, production of Ketones increases during fasting or when the intake of carbs falls below fifty grams in a day. When carbs are reduced or eliminated, Ketones can provide up to 70% of the brain's energy needs.

Gluconeogenesis

Even though most of the brain can utilize Ketones, there are portions that need glucose to function. On a diet that is low in carbs, some of the glucose may be supplied by the small number of carbs eaten. The rest originates from a process referred to as gluconeogenesis, which basically means making new glucose. During this process, the liver creates glucose for the brain to use. The glucose is manufactured using amino acids.

Furthermore, the liver can also make glucose from glycerol, the backbone that connects fatty acids and triglycerides. Because of gluconeogenesis, the brain will still get a steady supply of glucose even when carbs are low.

Ketogenic diet and epilepsy

Epilepsy is characterized by seizures that are connected to periods of over excitement within the brain cells. This disease causes uncontrolled jerking motions, loss of consciousness and mostly happens in children. Even though there are many medications for this condition, they are unable to control seizures in at least one-third of patients. Dr. Russell Wilder came up with the Ketogenic diet in 1921 to treat drug-resistant epilepsy in kids. This diet provides almost 100% of calories from fat and has been proven to copy the beneficial effects of starvation on seizures.

Ketogenic Diet Options for Epileptics

- The Classic Keto diet: 2-4% of calories from carbs, 6-10% from protein and 85-90% from fat.
- Modified Atkins diet: 4-6% of calories from carbs with mostly no restriction on protein. This diet allows 10g of carbs per day for children and 15g for adults.
- Medium-chain triglyceride Keto diet: initially, 20% carbs, 10% protein, 50% medium-chain triglycerides and 20% other fats.
- Low glycemic index treatment: limit carb choices to those with an index under 50. 20-30% of calories from protein, 10-20% from carbs and the remainder from fats.

The Keto Diet and Alzheimer's

Alzheimer's is the most common form of dementia. It is a disease in which the brain develops plaques and tangles that lead to memory loss. The brain cells become insulin resistant and are unable to properly use glucose leading to inflammation. Experts in brain health report that Alzheimer's disease has common features with epilepsy, including the same brain excitability that leads to seizures.

In a study of people with Alzheimer's, those who received an MCT supplement for three months had higher Ketone levels and a significant improvement in brain functionality as compared to a control group. Studies in animals also confirmed that the Keto diet is an effective way of fueling a brain that is affected by Alzheimer's.

The Keto diet also helps with congenital hyperinsulinism, migraine headaches, Parkinson's and traumatic brain injury. The ketogenic diet is also protective against brain injury and there are several studies to support this:

- A study conducted by George Washington University on 23 elderly people with mild cognitive impairment showed that a Keto diet improved verbal memory performance after 24 days as compared to a standard high carbohydrate diet. Moreover, in a placebo-controlled study, 152 patients with mild to moderate Alzheimer's disease were given either a Keto agent or a placebo, while maintaining a normal diet. Three months later, those who received the drug showed marked cognitive improvement compared to placebo, which was correlated with the level of Ketones in the blood.
- In another pilot study among seven Parkinson's patients, five were able to stick to the diet for 28 days and showed a marked reduction in their physical symptoms. In an animal model of Amyotrophic Lateral Sclerosis, a Keto diet also led to delayed motor neuron death and histological and functional improvements even though it did not increase lifespan.

Focus and Stress Relief

Lack of mental sharpness is a common symptom of an inadequate diet. This condition is called brain fog. The inability to recall information or to focus on a given task is usually as a result of this. Typically, there are two molecules that are involved in this area: GABA (gamma-Aminobutyric acid) and glutamate. GABA is the primary inhibitory neurotransmitter that reduces stimulation in the body while glutamate is the primary excitatory neurotransmitter that promotes stimulation.

Lack of focus and brain fog, among other things, are attributable to having too much glutamate and very little GABA. This happens when your brain has to utilize glutamate and glutamic acid for fuel leaving very little left over to be processed into GABA. When the brain only uses glutamate, it starts to over-process without a way to reduce stimulation.

Research shows that ketones are able to allow the additional glutamate to be efficiently processed into GABA. When you give the brain another form of energy by breaking down ketones, it is able to balance out the neurotransmitter production. This equilibrium increases GABA production thereby reducing the excess firing of neurons in the brain, causing better mental focus. Additionally, more GABA production in the brain has also been shown to help in the reduction of stress and anxiety. In order to boost your focus, try starting your day with a ketoproof coffee. The Medium Chain Triglycerides (MCTs) found inside of the coconut oil directly convert to ketones in the liver, offering you a significant boost of energy clarity during the day.

Increased Energy

Lack of energy is a familiar feeling for most people. As we strive to squeeze more time out of every day, we often find ourselves constantly running on fumes, almost nearing the end of our "tank." We gradually become more sluggish and fatigued and ultimately our mental performance and physical drive fail. However, the good news is that research has shown that those who follow a ketogenic diet can develop an increased mitochondrial function and a drop in free radicals.

The major role of mitochondria is to process the intake of food and oxygen and produce energy from that. This means that an increase in the mitochondrial function is equivalent to more energy for the cells leading to more energy for the body. Anyone who has switched to a ketogenic diet from a standard western diet will experience how their energy levels are stable throughout the day, no cravings for instant sugar, or caffeine, and no getting that mid-afternoon slump. Fat and the ketones derived from it are a readily available source of fuel. Once an individual is fat adapted and in ketosis, they will notice that they can easily go hours or even days without food and not experience extreme energy level swings.

Free radicals are formed when oxygen meets with certain molecules in the body. Free radicals are highly reactive and the danger comes from the damage they cause to the mitochondria. When this happens, cells may function poorly or even die. Reduction in the production of free radicals can lead to better cellular performance and better neurological stability causing more energy efficiency in the body. Therefore, instead of the body focusing on repairing the damage done by the free radicals, it can now focus on production of more energy.

Additionally, pairing the ketogenic diet with an exercise regimen will not only help boost mitochondrial function but also produce new mitochondria to help compensate increased energy demand.

Brain Function

Omega-3 and Omega-6 fatty acids are a critical part of the cognitive function in the body. These Omega Fatty Acids also play a pivotal role in the prevention of Non-Communicable Diseases such as heart disease. These Omega Fatty Acids are known as essential fatty acids meaning the body is not able to produce them on its own because our bodies lack the desaturase enzymes that are required for their production. Therefore, they must be consumed by direct supplementation or dietary intake. This is where the ketogenic diet comes in - a diet that is rich in fatty acids.

Studies have increasingly shown that the typical Western diet is significantly deficient in essential fatty acids, more particularly the Omega-3 fatty acids. Fatty acids comprise the majority of brain tissues and are also vital in the brain's function, exhibiting a direct link to sensory performance, learning, and memory. Studies have shown that there is a need to not only supplement our diet with essential fatty acids but also to maintain a suitable ratio of Omega-3 to Omega-6 fatty acids. Usually, we strive to aim at a ratio between 1:1 and 1:4 Omega 3s to Omega 6s- that is high on the ketogenic diet since consuming adequate amounts of healthy oils such as olive oil that contain balanced ratios of the fatty acids.

One study revealed that ketogenic diets even in the short term, can improve memory function in older adults. A ketogenic diet was also shown to increase ATP concentrations and that the number of hippocampal mitochondria in the brain of mice grew up by up to 50%. The hippocampus is involved in learning, memory, and emotion. Dr. Myhill, a researcher in the study, stated that the brain and the heart run at least 25% more efficiently on ketones than on glucose.

Brain Mitochondrial Biogenesis

Ketogenic diets help upregulate mitochondrial biogenesis in the brain. It creates new power plants in the brain which are effective in burning fat-derived fuel. This regulation is useful for the anticonvulsant benefits in patients with epilepsy and also in other brain disorders with glucose uptake challenges. By supplying an alternative source of brain power, brains which do not operate so well on glucose can start burning fat.

There are reasons to believe that ketone-induced mitochondrial biogenesis in the brain improves brain functions since the extra energy sources help improve how the brain works. Additionally, exercise helps to increase blood flow to the brain, provides more oxygen and energy and also reduces free radical damage and memory enhancement. Exercise stimulates the creation of new neurons and the production of brain-derived neurotrophic factor (BDNF, which is a chemical that is useful in neuron preservation and its formation. Exercise also boosts gene expression that promotes plasticity, the brain's vital power to alter neural pathways.

The mitochondria work much more efficiently on a ketogenic diet since they are able to increase energy levels in an efficient, stable, long-burning and steady way. A ketogenic diet induces epigenetic changes that increase the energetic output of the mitochondria, lowers the production of damaging free radicals and enhances the production of GABA. Mitochondria are tailored to use fat for energy. When the mitochondria use fat as a source as energy, its toxic load is decreased, the expression of energy producing genes are lowered, and the inflammatory energetic-end-products load is decreased.

Fat metabolism and the generation of ketone bodies that include beta-hydroxybutyrate and acetoacetate by the liver can only take place within the mitochondria, leaving chemicals within the cell but outside the mitochondria readily available to enhance potent anti-inflammatory antioxidants. The ultimate key to optimal health is the status of our mitochondria. While it is true that some individuals may need extra support in form of nutritional supplements in order to heal these much-needed energy factories, the diet remains the ultimate key for proper equilibrium.

Our bodies need energy in order to perform its functions. This energy comes in the form of ATP that is mainly produced by the mitochondria. Cells in some parts of the body have more mitochondria than other parts and this reflects the amount of energy that they need in order to properly function. The brain is one of the areas that require more energy in order to function properly. By improving the number and the energetic output in the brain, a significant amount of energy is supplied to the brain. This is what provides much of the brain-boosting benefits. Ketogenic diet and fasting are some of the most promising methods for regulating mitochondrial biogenesis.

Anti-Seizure Effect

A classic ketogenic diet has three major components. One, it is calorie restricted which has the effect of reducing seizure frequency in people who get them and also increases longevity. Second, the ketogenic diet is acidic. Ketones or fats affect ATP sensitive $K+$ ion channels, making hyperpolarization easier to maintain. The extra protons block proton-sensitive ion channels, the ketone bodies, or fat themselves, can affect the neuron membranes thereby making them harder to excite. Third, ketones lower glucose levels. Lower glucose levels are linked to a higher seizure threshold and less neuronal excitability.

Clearing Brain Fog

Increased ammonia levels and decreased GABA levels lead to a condition called "brain fog". The synapses fire blanks, the neuronal communication medium is cold molasses, therefore, work suffers, no task gets done. According to a study by Dr. Bill Lagakos, ketosis has the potential to reduce brain fog. Ketosis upregulates GABA signaling. GABA opposes glutamate, the excitatory neurotransmitter. Glutamate is useful in cognitive function but too much of it can lead to neuronal injury and neurodegeneration. GABA is the counterpoise.

Brain-Derived Neurotrophic Factor

Abbreviated as BDNF, its main function involves regulating the growth of neural connections in the brain. Low levels of BDNF have been associated with mental disorders such as depression, Alzheimer's, schizophrenia, and Huntington's disease, making it a target for modern medical research. It is believed that fasting or a fasting-mimicking diet such as a ketogenic diet has the ability to improve neurodegenerative disorders by upregulating brain-derived neurotrophic factor, BDNF. This upregulation of BDNF combats neurodegeneration by augmenting the continued growth and development of neuronal connections.

Less Oxidative Stress

Whereas oxidative stress is beneficial in small amounts, in excess it can be damaging to your cell's mitochondria. Excessive oxidative stress creates hampered mitochondrial output and inflammation. Since oxidative stress cause damage to the mitochondrial, it has a negative impact on every cell in the body. In addition, because the brain is so reliant on healthy mitochondria, it is often the first to suffer the effects of oxidative stress.

Oxidative stress occurs as a natural byproduct of energy production in the mitochondria. The metabolism of ketones has been shown to produce much lower levels of oxidative stress as compared to glucose metabolism, thereby lowering inflammation and augmenting mitochondrial health. In the end, this results in improved energy production.

Neurodegenerative disorders that are characterized by demyelination. For instance, multiple sclerosis is thought to be largely influenced by chronic inflammation, making the ketogenic diet a desirable therapy.

Improved Insulin Signaling

Most people today are probably burning sugar as their primary source of fuel. In order for the sugar to enter the cells to be converted into ATP, it requires insulin for its transportation. As a result of chronic high carbohydrate consumption, many individuals develop undesirable blood sugar regulation that often starts with a spike in sugar levels and ends with a rapid crash.

This imbalance in blood glucose is highly damaging to the brain and can be clearly observed in instances of congenital hyperinsulinism. A ketogenic diet has been shown to boost insulin signaling and lower the side effects linked to this rollercoaster blood sugar pattern.

Omega-3 Favoring

Most individuals today following a standard American diet have increased intakes of oxidized omega-6 fatty acids and very little omega -3 fatty acids from pasteurized meats and fish. Omega-6 fatty acids are used in the eicosanoid pathway in the body which is critical for producing inflammation. Whereas temporary inflammation is helpful for the stimulation of the healing process in the body, an excessive omega-6 level can lead to chronic inflammation which only causes more problems. Ketogenic diets include adequate healthy fats that help bring the ratio of omega-3 to omega- fatty acids back to equilibrium and help reduce inflammation. Increasing the ratio of omega-3 to omega-6 fatty acids can reduce the risk of cancer and improve brain function.

Glutamate GABA Balance

As we've discussed GABA and glutamate are two very important neurotransmitters that are instrumental in your focus. Adequate neurological functions require a balanced interplay between these two neurotransmitters.

An imbalance in these two neurotransmitters is usually evident as an excess of glutamate. This has been linked to brain disorders such as epilepsy, autism, Lou Gehrig's, Amyotrophic Lateral Sclerosis and mood disorders. In addition, individuals with excess and very low GABA levels tend to feel anxious, have difficulty sleeping, and experience brain fog. In a healthy individual, excess glutamate is converted into GABA to help balance the neural processes. Chronically increased glutamate is highly inflammatory since it incessantly overstimulates brain cells. Following a ketogenic diet has been shown to increase focus and lowers levels of anxiety and stress

Chapter Summary

This chapter went in depth to discuss:

- The benefits of the ketogenic diet and the science behind them
- Dangers of the Ketogenic diet
- Ketones
- Getting into ketosis

In the next chapter, you will learn about some of the Ketogenic diet eating plans.

Chapter Nine: Ketogenic Eating Plans and Recipe Ideas

There are several versions of the ketogenic diet:

- Standard ketogenic diet: this is a very low carb, moderate protein, and high-fat diet. It consists of 75% fat, 20% protein, and 5% carbohydrates.
- Cyclical ketogenic diet: this diet is about periods of higher carb intake such as five ketogenic days succeeded by two days of high carb foods.
- Targeted ketogenic diet: this diet allows one to add carbohydrates when working out
- High protein ketogenic diet: this is the same as the standard ketogenic diet but it contains more protein. The ratio is 60% fat, 35% protein, and 5% carbohydrates

It is important to note that only the standard and high protein ketogenic diets have been studied thoroughly. Cyclical and targeted ketogenic diets are methods that are more advanced and primarily used by athletes and bodybuilders. Of all these diets, the standard ketogenic diet is the most known and recommended.

There are also crockpot recipes for the Ketogenic diet. A crockpot, also known as a slow cooker, is a countertop electrical appliance that is used to simmer or cook food at low temperatures. It is a multi-purpose kitchen appliance that allows you to cook soups, stews, pot roast, casseroles, and even desserts.

The Crockpot comes with a heating component that keeps a steady temperature between 80⁰C and 95⁰C. The Crockpot comes with a lid that enables condensation inside the Crockpot. Also, the condensation from within the pot transmits heat properly within its walls so food is cooked all through.

To use a Crockpot, take the raw food and liquid in the form of stock or water inside the Crockpot. Food is cooked at temperatures of between 70⁰C and 80⁰C. It's good to try out a crockpot if you never have- because the food isn't cooked at the boiling point, it retains more nutrients and enzymes as compared to when it's cooked conventionally.

Advantages of Crockpots
Crockpots are very popular kitchen applications. They are heaven-sent to busy people as you can cook your foods while you are out so that they are ready by the time you are ready to eat. But more than suitability, there are also many aids to using Crockpots. Below are the advantages of using Crockpots when cooking your food.

- **They are better for cooking inexpensive cuts of meat:** Meats that come with connective tissues are cooked better in slow cookers. They can be stewed to create tastier dishware. By using Crockpots, you can make delightful meals without the need to buy costly cuts of meat.

- **Food does not burn:** Since food is cooked using low temperature, it does not burn even if it has been cooking for a long time.
- **Brings out the full flavor of food:** Food cooked in low temperature for a long time tends to have better flavor than those cooked in conventional systems. Thus, if you are cooking casseroles, stews, soups, and one-pot meals, they taste better than if they are cooked on the stovetop.
- **Uses less electricity:** A Crockpot does not consume too much electricity when cooking food so you can save on your electric bill even if it is running for a long time.

Because the crockpot is so beneficial, here are sample crockpot recipes to get you started:

BREAKFAST

1. Crockpot Pumpkin Coconut Breakfast Bars

Preparation Time: 20 Minutes

Serves: 8

Ingredients
- 1 ¾ cup canned pumpkin puree
- 2/3 cup swerve sweetener
- 1 teaspoon raw apple cider vinegar

- 3 eggs, beaten
- 1 cup coconut flour
- 1 tablespoon pumpkin pie spice
- ½ tablespoon cinnamon
- ½ teaspoon baking soda
- ¼ teaspoon salt
- 1/3 cup pecan, toasted and chopped

Directions

1. Line the bottom of the Crockpot with parchment paper that has been lightly oiled with cooking oil.

2. In a bowl, mix the pumpkin puree, sweetener, apple cider vinegar, and eggs.

3. In another bowl, mix the coconut flour, pumpkin pie spice, cinnamon, baking soda, and salt.

4. Pour the wet ingredients to the dry ingredients and fold until well mixed.

5. Pour the batter into the Crockpot and sprinkle with pecans.

6. Cover with lid. Cook for 3 hours on low or until a toothpick can come out clean.

Nutrition information: Calories per serving:187.4; Carbohydrates: 8.5g; Protein: 6g; Fat: 17.2g; Sugar: 2.5g; Sodium: 165 mg; Fiber: 3g

2. Overnight Eggs Benedict Casserole

Preparation Time: 25 Minutes

Serves: 10

Ingredients

- 1-pound Canadian bacon, sliced
- 10 large eggs, beaten
- 1 cup milk
- Salt and pepper to taste
- 6 egg yolks
- 2 tablespoons chives, chopped
- 1 ½ sticks butter, cubed

Directions

1. Spray cooking oil in the Crockpot's ceramic interior.

2. Take the bacon slices at the bottom of the Crockpot.

3. In a bowl, mix the eggs and milk. Season with salt and pepper to taste.

4. Pour over the bacon.

5. Close the lid and cook for 1 ½ hours.

6. Open the lid and Take the egg yolks on top. Sprinkle with chopped chives.

7. Continue cooking for another 1 ½ hours or until the egg mixture is done.

8. While still warm, keep butter on top.

Nutrition information: Calories per serving: 256; Carbohydrates: 2g; Protein: 16.2g; Fat: 21g; Sugar: 0g; Sodium: 734 mg; Fiber: 0.3g

3. Crustless Crockpot Spinach Quiche

Preparation Time: 50 Minutes

Serves: 6

Ingredients

- · 1 tablespoon ghee
- · 2 cups baby Bella mushrooms, chopped
- · 1 medium red bell peppers, sliced
- · 1 package chopped spinach, drained
- · 8 eggs, beaten
- · 1 cup sour cream

- ½ teaspoon salt
- ¼ teaspoon black pepper
- 1 ½ cup cheddar cheese, shredded
- 2 tablespoons chives, chopped
- ½ cup almond flour
- ¼ teaspoon baking soda

Directions

1. Oil the slow cooker with cooking spray.

2. In a skillet, heat the ghee and sauté the mushrooms and bell peppers for 4 hours. Add the kale and cook for another minute. Set aside.

3. In a bowl, mix the eggs and sour cream. Season with salt and pepper. Stir in the cheese and chives. Add the almond flour and baking soda. Mix until well mixed. Stir in the vegetable mixture.

4. Pour the mixture in the Crockpot and cook on low for 5 hours or 3 hours on high.

Nutrition information: Calories per serving: 383.1; Carbohydrates: 7.3g; Protein: 15.1g; Fat:18g; Sugar: 0g; Sodium: 547 mg; Fiber: 3.2g

LUNCH

1. Crockpot Beef Roast

Preparation Time: 20 Minutes

Serves: 6

Ingredients

- 2-pounds beef chuck roast, trimmed of excess fat

- 1 ½ teaspoons salt

- ¾ teaspoon black pepper

- 2 tablespoons fresh basil, chopped

- 1 large yellow onion, chopped

- 4 cloves of garlic, minced

- 2 bay leaves

- 2 cups beef stock

Directions

1. Pat the beef roast dry with a paper towel and rub with salt, pepper, and chopped basil.

2. Add the roast to the Crockpot and spread the onion, garlic, and bay leaves.

3. Pour the beef stock over everything.

4. Close the lid and cook on low for 10 hours until tender.

Nutrition information: Calories per serving: 234; Carbohydrates: 2.4g; Protein: 33.1g; Fat: 10.3g; Sugar: 0.9g; Sodium: 758.2mg; Fiber: 0.5g

2. Chipotle Barbecue Chicken

Preparation Time: 20 Minutes

Serves: 5

Ingredients

· ¼ cup water

· 1 14-ounce boneless chicken breasts, skin removed

· 1 14-ounce boneless chicken thighs, skin removed

· Salt and pepper to taste

· 2 tablespoons chipotle Tabasco sauce

· 1 onion, chopped

· 4 tablespoons unsalted butter

- 1 cup tomato sauce

- 1/3 cup apple cider vinegar

- ½ cup water

- 2 tablespoons yellow mustard

- ¼ teaspoon garlic powder

Directions

1. Add all ingredients to your Crockpot.

2. Give everything a stir so that the chicken is coated with the sauce.

3. Close the lid and cook on low for 8 hours.

Nutrition information: Calories per serving: 482; Carbohydrates: 3g; Protein: 29.4g; Fat: 18.7g; Sugar: 0g; Sodium: 462mg; Fiber: 0.3g

3. Spicy Shredded Chicken Lettuce Wraps
Preparation Time: 15 Minutes

Serves: 8

Ingredients

- 4 chicken breast, skin and bones removed

- 1 cup tomato salsa

- 1 teaspoon onion powder

- 1 can diced green chilies

- 1 tablespoon Tabasco sauce

- 2 tablespoons lime juice, freshly squeezed

- Salt and pepper to taste

- 2 large heads iceberg lettuce, rinsed

Directions

1. Take the chicken breast in the Crockpot.

2. Pour over the tomato salsa, onion powder, green chilies, Tabasco sauce, and lime juice. Season with salt and pepper to taste.

3. Close the lid and cook for 10 hours.

4. Shred the chicken meat using a fork.

5. Take on top of lettuce leaves.

6. Garnish with sour cream, tomatoes, or avocado slices if needed.

Nutrition information: Calories per serving: 231; Carbohydrates: 3g; Protein: 23g; Fat: 12g; Sugar: 0.5g; Sodium: 375mg; Fiber: 2g

4. Bacon Cheeseburger Casserole

Preparation Time: 50 Minutes

Serves: 8

Ingredients

· 2-pounds ground beef

· ½ onion, sliced thinly

· ½ teaspoon salt

· ½ teaspoon black pepper

· 1 15-ounce can cream of mushroom soup

· 1 15-ounce can cheddar cheese soup

· ½ pounds bacon, cooked and crumbled

· 2 cups cheddar cheese, grated

Directions

1. Brown the ground beef and onions in a skillet over medium heat. Season with salt and pepper to taste.

2. Take the beef in the Crockpot and add the cream of mushroom soup and cheese soup.

3. Pour in the bacon and half of your cheddar cheese. Give a stir.

4. Cook on low for 4 hours.

5. An hour before the cooking time is over, add the remaining cheese on top.

Nutrition information: Calories per serving: 322; Carbohydrates: 2g; Protein: 36g; Fat: 21g; Sugar: 0g; Sodium: 271mg; Fiber: 1.3g

DINNER

1. Bacon Cheddar Broccoli Salad

Preparation Time: 35 Minutes

Serves: 6

Ingredients

- 6 slices raw bacon, chopped
- 1 bunch steamed broccoli, cut into small florets
- ¾ cup mayonnaise

- 2 tablespoons apple cider vinegar

- 3 packets stevia powder

- ½ cup cheddar cheese

- ¼ cup onion, chopped

- ¼ cup sunflower seeds, roasted

Directions

1. Put a parchment paper on the bottom of the Crockpot. Add the bacon to the Crockpot.

2. Cook on low for 8 hours or until the bacon is crispy.

3. Add the bacon to a bowl and add the steamed broccoli.

4. In another bowl, add the mayonnaise, apple cider vinegar, and stevia powder. Mix until well mixed.

5. Pour over the bacon and broccoli and toss to mix.

6. Add the cheddar cheese, onion, and sunflower seeds.

Nutrition information: Calories per serving: 231; Carbohydrates: 8.1g; Protein: 16g; Fat: 15.3g; Sugar: 2.4g; Sodium: 751mg; Fiber: 3g

2. Chicken Yellow Curry

Preparation Time: 40 Minutes

Serves: 6

Ingredients

- 1 ½ pounds chicken breasts, skin and bones removed
- 6 cups mixed vegetables (preferably broccoli, and cauliflower)
- 1 can full-fat coconut milk
- 1 cup crushed tomatoes
- 1 tablespoon cumin
- 2 teaspoons ground coriander
- 2 teaspoons ground ginger
- 2 teaspoons ground ginger powder
- 1 teaspoon cinnamon
- ½ teaspoon cayenne pepper
- 1 cup water
- Salt to taste

Directions

1. Take the chicken and vegetables in the Crockpot.

2. Add the rest of the ingredients and stir to mix everything.

3. Close the lid and cook on low for 6 hours.

Nutrition information: Calories per serving: 425; Carbohydrates: 3g; Protein: 23g; Fat: 31.4g; Sugar: 0g; Sodium: 371.4mg; Fiber:0.9g

3. Thai Whole Chicken Soup

Preparation Time: 25 Minutes

Serves: 10

Ingredients

- 1 whole chicken

- 1 stalk lemongrass, cut into chunks

- 20 fresh basil leaves

- 5 thick slices of ginger

- 1 tablespoon salt or more if needed

- 1 lime, sliced

Directions

1. Put the whole chicken inside the Crockpot.

2. Surround it with lemongrass stalks, 10 basil leaves, and ginger.

3. Fill the Crockpot with water until the maximum line. Season with salt.

4. Cook on low for 10 hours or until the chicken is tender.

5. Serve with lime and the remaining basil leaves.

Nutrition information: Calories per serving: 475; Carbohydrates: 2g; Protein: 42g; Fat: 12g; Sugar: 0g; Sodium: 278 mg; Fiber:0.5g

As you can see these are very easy recipes. With only a little bit of planning, you could be eating very well while experiencing the full benefits of the keto diet. Here is what your week could like on a seven-day keto diet plan, it's both very filling and very tasty:

Day one

Breakfast:

A serving of Keto Brunch Spread

Macros:

Fat-38g   Protein- 17g   Carbs- 3g Calories- 426

Lunch:

A serving of crispy skin salmon with pesto cauliflower rice

Macros:

Fat- 51g Protein- 34g Carbs- 10g   Calories- 647

Dinner:

A serving of superfood meatballs and keto creamed spinach

Macros:

Fat-36g   Protein- 36g   Carbs- 7g   Calories- 485

Total daily macros:

Fat-125g   Protein- 87g Carbs- 20g   Calories- 1,558

Day two:

Breakfast:

A serving of chocolate pancakes with blueberry butter

Macros:

Fat-50g   Protein- 27g   Carbs- 11.5g   Calories-611

Lunch

A serving of turkey sausage frittata, four slices of bacon fried in a tablespoon of butter and a cup of coffee or tea with MCT oil powder

Macros:

Fat- 50g   Protein- 25   Carbs- 5.5   Calories- 572

Dinner:

A serving of lemon herb low carb keto meatloaf

Macros:

Fat-29g   Protein- 33g   Carbs- 2g   Calories- 344

Daily macros:

Fat- 129g   Protein- 85g   Carbs-19g   Calories-1,527g

Day three

Breakfast

A serving of bacon, egg and cheese breakfast casserole

Macros:

Fat- 38g   Protein-43g   Carbs- 2g   Calories- 437

Lunch

A serving of white turkey chili with 2 cups of mixed leafy greens and 1 tablespoon of olive oil

Macros:

Fat- 44.5g   Protein- 28.8g   Carbs- 5.5g Calories- 568

Dinner:

A serving of Portobello bun cheeseburger, celeriac oven fries, and homemade keto mayo

Macros:

Fat- 40g   Protein- 31g   Carbs- 13g   Calories- 539

Daily macros:

Fat- 122.5g   Protein- 102.8g   Carbs- 20.5g Calories- 1,544

Day four

Breakfast

A serving of Keto power breakfast (really, this is anything you want that does not exceed the recommended macros below)

Macros:

Fat- 27g Protein-10.5g Carbs- 7g Calories- 305

Lunch

A serving of crispy cheesy chicken salad

Macros:

Fat- 36.5g Protein- 55g Carbs- 8g Calories- 575

Dinner

4oz grilled ribeye steak, two tablespoons of grass-fed butter and two cups of mixed leafy greens with a tablespoon of avocado oil and salt

Macros:

Fat- 62g Protein-20g Carbs-1g Calories- 636

Dessert

MCT(Medium-chain Triglyceride) fat bomb

Macros:

Fat- 8g   Protein-1g   Carbs- 2g   Calories-81

Daily macros:

Fat- 133.5g   Protein-86.5g   Carbs-18g   Calories-1,597

Day five

Breakfast

Avocado breakfast bowl

Macros:

Fat- 40g   Protein- 25g   Carbs- 3g   Calories-500

Lunch

A serving of roasted chicken stacks

Macros:

Fat- 25g   Protein- 34g   Carbs-5.5g   Calories- 369

Dinner:

A serving of cheesy broccoli meatza

Macros:

Fat- 24g Protein-32g Carbs-7g Calories-375

Dessert

Two servings of macadamia nut fat bomb

Macros:

Fat-34g Protein-2g Carbs- 4g Calories- 200

Daily macros:

Fat- 123g Protein- 93g Carbs- 19.5g Calories- 1,444

Day six

Breakfast

Low carb acai almond butter smoothie

Macros:

Fat-20g Protein- 15g Carbs-6g Calories-345

Lunch

A serving of keto beef bulgogi

Macros:

Fat-18g Protein- 25g Carbs-3g Calories- 242

Snack

A hard-boiled egg with an ounce of almonds

Macros:

Fat-19g Protein-12g Carbs-3g Calories-241

Dinner

A serving of creamy mushroom chicken

Macros:

Fat- 27g Protein-24g Carbs-3g Calories-334

Dessert

Keto chocolate mousse

Macros:

Fat-14g Protein-17.5g Carbs-6g Calories-248

Daily macros:

Fat- 98g Protein- 93.5g Carbs-21g Calories-1,410

Day seven

Breakfast

Keto bulletproof coffee

Macros:

Fat-31g Protein- 1g Carbs- 0.5g Calories-280

Lunch

A serving of low carb crispy keto fried chicken with a cup of steamed broccoli

Macros:

Fat-27g Protein-33.5g Carbs-6.5g Calories-494

Dinner

A serving of low carb keto lasagna

Macros:

Fat-21g Protein-32g Carbs-12g Calories-364

Snack/dessert

Collagen mug cake

Macros:

Fat-43.5g Protein-27g Carbs-4g Calories-535

Daily macros:

Fat-122.5g Protein-93.5g Carbs-23g Calories-1,673

It is important for you to note that it will not be possible to get the numbers right every day. However, it's better to stay under instead of above your calorie count when it comes to your protein and carb intake because if they are excessive, you will get out of ketosis.

You now have an idea of what your days on keto can look like, let me take you through the basics of planning your own meals. Let's have a look at the keto foods by grouping them into categories:

Saturated and Monosaturated Fats

·   Grass-fed butter or ghee

·   Olive oil

·   Macadamia nuts

·   Coconut oil

·   Almonds

·   Seeds like chia and hemp

- Avocados

- Fatty fish

- Egg yolks

Proteins

- Grass-fed beef

- Poultry

- Pork

- Fish

- Shellfish

- Eggs

- Lamb and goat

- Organ meats

Always avoid processed meats as they may contain added sugars, suspect ingredients, or even sauces. You may be ignorantly increasing your sugar and carb intake.

Veggies

- Kale

- Bell peppers

- Asparagus

- Spinach

- Celery

- Swiss chard

- Cucumber

- Bok choy

- Romaine lettuce

- Zucchini

- Radish

- Arugula

- Cauliflower

- Brussels sprouts

- Mushroom and broccoli

Fruits

It is important to eat fruits in small portions because of their high sugar content. You can choose fruits with low sugar such as:

- Strawberries

- Raspberries

- Cranberries

- Blackberries

- Blueberries

When it comes to fruits and veggies, it is okay to have either frozen or fresh, but organic is best even though it is not a must.

Dairy Products

Most dairy products are allowed in the keto diet. It is actually advisable to choose the full-fat dairy products because the low-fat ones tend to add sugar even when they cut fat.

- Hard cheeses like cheddar and swiss

- Heavy cream

- Full-fat yogurts

- Soft cheese like brie and bleu cheese

- Sour cream

- Cottage cheese

- Cream cheese

Condiments, Spices, and Sweeteners

Homemade is recommended because you have the power to control the sugar quantity.

- Soy sauce

- Yellow mustard

- Ketchup with no added sugar

- Sauerkraut with no added sugar

- Horseradish

Herbs and Spices

To be safe, stick to dried herbs and spices.

- Basil

- Cumin

- Cinnamon

- Nutmeg

- Turmeric

- Garlic

- Oregano

- Rosemary

- Parsley

- Thyme

- Lemon juices

- Cilantro

- Salt and pepper

- Chili powder

- Cayenne pepper

Sweeteners

When choosing sweeteners, keep two things in mind: Always use low glycemic index sweeteners as they will not affect your blood sugar levels or influence your carb intake, and steer clear of sugar alcohol-based sweeteners as they cause bloating and gas

- Stevia

- Erythritol

- Monk fruit

Supplements

The aim of exogenous ketone supplements is to provide the body with additional ketones, which, again, is energy. These supplements enable you to get into ketosis at any time instead of having to wait for days for the diet to completely kick in. They can be taken in between meals or before a workout session.

MCT Oils and Powders

MCT is an acronym for medium chain triglyceride. They are meant to help the body burn fat instead of carbs. They are effective in losing weight, energy, and digestion. You can choose between MCT oil powder, liquid C8 MCT oil or MCT oil capsules depending on what works well for you.

Collagen Protein Supplements

Of all the thousands of proteins in our bodies, collagen is the most abundant one, it accounts for 30% of all the body's protein. It is like a glue that holds our body together.

Micronutrient Supplements

When you are on keto, you will have to cut down on many starchy fruits and veggies. Consequently, you will be deficient in vitamins, nutrients, and antioxidants that these carb-rich foods offer. Keto microgreen supplements are the solution to this problem as they contain:

- Greens and a vegetable blend of raw and organic veggies
- Fruit and berry mix of raw and organic berry fruits

- MCT powder made from coconut oil. It helps your body absorb vitamins and minerals from the greens and fruits.
- Liver support and digestion enzymes. They assist you in getting the most out of the micronutrient blend by making sure that everything is absorbed and utilized by the body.

Chapter Summary

This chapter talked about:

- Different versions of the Ketogenic diet
- Ketogenic crockpot recipes
- A sample 7-day meal plan
- Ketogenic Food Group breakdowns and diet supplements

In the next chapter, you will read through some delicious Ketogenic recipes.

Chapter Ten: Ketogenic Diet Recipes

This is by no means an exhaustive recipe list, but you can use this chapter as your go-to cookbook when you get started on your ketogenic diet.

Breakfast Recipes

Ketogenic White Pizza Frittata (8 servings)

Nutrient intake per serving; Carbs: 2.1g, Fat: 23.8g, Protein: 19.4g, Calories: 298

These are great when microwaved, reheated in the oven, or just plain cold. This recipe makes use of different cheeses in the frittata base and is topped with a mozzarella and pepperoni combo. Inside you'll find spinach which makes sure we get some greens first thing in the morning. The texture is a bit more on the dense side for a frittata due to the melted ricotta and parmesan cheese inside.

Ingredients

- Twelve large eggs
- 9 oz. bag of frozen spinach
- 1 oz. pepperoni

- 5 oz. mozzarella cheese

- One teaspoon of minced garlic

- Half a cup of fresh ricotta cheese

- Half a cup of parmesan cheese

- Four tablespoons of olive oil

- A quarter teaspoon of nutmeg

- Salt and pepper

Preparation:

- Place the frozen spinach into the microwave for between 3-4 minutes or until defrosted. It should not be hot. Squeeze the spinach using your hands and drain as much water as you can. Set it aside.

- Preheat oven to 375F. Mix the eggs, olive oil, and spices. Whisk until properly mixed.

- Add in the ricotta cheese, parmesan cheese, and spinach. Break the spinach into small pieces using your hands while adding.

- Pour the mixture into a cast iron skillet then sprinkle mozzarella cheese on the top. Add pepperoni on top of that.

·   Bake it for half an hour. In case you are using a glass container in place of cast iron, bake it for 45 minutes or until it is completely set.

·   Slice it up and devour it. You can top it up using crème Fraiche, ranch dressing, or your favorite fatty sauce.

Ketogenic Brownie Muffins (a serving of 6)

Nutrient intake per serving; Carbs: 3.3g, Fat: 13.4g, Protein: 7g, Calories: 183

These breakfast muffins are rich, hearty, and moist. They are also low in carbs and high in fibers because of their flaxseed base and wholesome ingredients. Each muffin offers a rich and dark taste of chocolate with a hint of caramel. These muffins are satisfying and can keep you full until lunch hour. They're also easy to make!

Ingredients

·   A cup of golden flaxseed meal

·   A quarter cup of cocoa powder

·   A tablespoon of cinnamon

·   Half a tablespoon of baking powder

·   Half a teaspoon of salt

·   A large egg

- Two tablespoons of coconut oil

- A quarter cup of sugar-free caramel syrup

- Half a cup of pumpkin puree

- A teaspoon of vanilla extract

- A teaspoon of apple cider vinegar

- A quarter cup of slivered almonds

Method of preparation:

- Preheat the oven to 350F and mix all the dry ingredients in a mixing bowl

- In a different bowl, mix all the wet ingredients

- You then pour all the wet ingredients into the dry ingredients and mix well

- Line a muffin tin with paper liners and spoon about a quarter cup of batter into each liner. Sprinkle the slivered almonds over each muffin and gently press for them to stick.

- Bake in the oven for a quarter of an hour.

- Enjoy when warm or cool

Ketogenic lemon poppy seed muffins (12 servings)

Nutrient intake per serving; Carbs: 1.5g, Fat: 11.3g, Protein: 3.7g, Calories: 129

These muffins take little time to make and store. They contain 1.5g net carbs per muffin. When fresh, their bottoms crust up well and add an extra crunch when they come out of the oven.

Ingredients

- 3/4 of a cup of blanched almond flour
- 1/4 cup of golden flaxseed meal
- 1/3 of a cup of erythritol
- 1 tablespoon of baking powder
- 2 tablespoons of poppy seeds
- 1/4 cup of salted butter that is melted
- 1/4 cup of heavy cream
- 3 large eggs
- Zest of two lemons
- 3 tablespoons of lemon juice
- 1 tablespoon of vanilla extract
- 25 drops of liquid stevia

Method of preparation

- Preheat the oven to 350 F. In a bowl, use a fork to mix the almond flour, flaxseed meal, erythritol and poppy seeds.

- Stir in the melted butter, eggs, and the heavy cream until smooth. Make sure that there are no lumps in the batter

- Once it becomes smooth, add in the baking powder, liquid stevia, vanilla extract, lemon zest, and lemon juice. Mix thoroughly

- Divide the batter equally among 12 cupcake molds.

- Bake for twenty minutes or until they slightly turn brown.

- Remove from the oven and let it cool for ten minutes

Bacon cheddar chive omelet (one serving)

Nutrient intake per serving; Carbs: 1g, Fat: 39g, Protein: 24g, Calories: 463

The bacon offers a burst of flavor with the eggs and cheese, as well as providing more protein. The chives offer a delicious sweet onion taste.

Ingredients

- Two slices of cooked bacon

- A teaspoon of bacon fat

- Two large eggs

- 1 oz. of cheddar cheese

- Two stalks chives

- Salt and pepper

Preparation:

- Ensure that you have all the ingredients ready because the omelet cooks quite fast. Shred the cheese, precook the bacon and chop the chives

- Heat a pan with bacon fat in it at a medium-low heat. Add the eggs then season with chives, salt, and pepper.

- As soon as the edges start to set, add the bacon to the center and let it cook for around thirty seconds longer. You then turn off the heat

- Add the cheese on top the bacon and make sure it's centered. You then take two edges of the omelet and fold them onto the cheese. Hold the edges for a moment as the cheese partially melts to act as an adhesive to hold them in place.

- Do the same with the other edges creating a burrito of sorts. You then flip it over and let it cook for a little longer in the warm pan

·   Serve with extra cheese, bacon, and chives if you like.

Ketogenic breakfast burger (two servings)

Nutrient intake per serving; Carbs: 3g, Fat: 56g, Protein: 30.5g, Calories: 655

This is a good option for either a brunch or heavier breakfast. This especially good when you know you'll have an active day.

Ingredients

·   4 oz. sausage

·   2 oz. pepper jack cheese

·   4 slices of bacon

·   2 large eggs

·   A tablespoon of butter

·   A tablespoon of PB (peanut butter) fit powder

·   Salt and pepper

Preparation

·   Begin by cooking the bacon. Lay the strips on a wire rack over a cookie sheet. Bake at 400F for 25 minutes or until crisp.

- Mix together butter and PB fit powder in a small container to rehydrate. Set aside

- Form sausage patties and cook in a pan over medium to high heat. Turn over when the bottom side is browned

- Grate the cheese and have it ready

- When the other side of the sausage patty is browned, add the cheese and cover with a lid

- Remove the sausage patties and melted cheese and set aside. Fry an egg in the same pan

- Bring everything together; sausage patty, egg, bacon and the rehydrated PB fit on top.

LUNCH RECIPES

Broccoli chicken zucchini boats (2 servings)

Nutrient intake per serving; Carbs: 5g, Fat: 34g, Protein: 30g, Calories: 500

This is the perfect lunch when you want to have something a little out of the ordinary. The fillings are incredibly flavorful and satisfying.

Ingredients

- 10 oz. zucchini

- 2 tablespoons of butter

- 3 oz. shredded cheddar cheese

- A cup of broccoli

- 6 oz. shredded rotisserie chicken

- 2 tablespoons of sour cream

- A stalk of green onion

- Salt and pepper

Preparation

- Preheat the oven to 400F and cut the zucchini into halves, lengthwise.

- Using a spoon, scoop out most of the zucchini until you are left with a shell that is about a centimeter thick

- Pour a tablespoon of melted butter into each zucchini boat and season with salt or pepper and place in the oven. This gives zucchini time to cook as you prepare the filling. This takes about twenty minutes

- Shred your chicken using two forks to pull the meat apart. Measure out 6oz. and place the rest in the refrigerator for another meal.

- Cut up your broccoli florets until they are bite-sized

·   Mix the chicken and broccoli with sour cream to keep them moist and creamy. Season.

·   As soon as the zucchini has cooked, take them out, add the chicken and broccoli filling

·   Sprinkle cheddar cheese on top of your chicken and broccoli and pop them back into the oven for another 15 minutes until the cheese is melted and browning

·   Garnish with chopped green onion

Cheese Stuffed Bacon Wrapped Hot Dogs (6 hot dogs)

Nutrient intake per serving; Carbs: 0.3g, Fat: 34.5g, Protein: 16.8g, Calories: 380

This recipe is especially great because it only takes about 10 minutes to prepare.

Ingredients

·   Six hot dogs

·   12 slices of bacon

·   2 oz. cheddar cheese

·   Half a teaspoon of garlic powder

·   Half a teaspoon of onion powder

- Salt and pepper

How to prepare

- Heat the oven to 400F. Slit all the hotdogs to create space for cheese.

- Slice 2oz. cheddar cheese into small and long rectangles. Stuff them into the hotdogs.

- Tightly wrap one slice of bacon around the hotdog

- Go on and tightly wrap the second slice of bacon around the hotdog. Make sure it slightly overlaps with the first slice.

- Poke each side of the bacon and hotdog with a toothpick and secure the bacon in place.

- Then set it on a wire rack that's on top of a cookie sheet. Season with garlic powder, onion powder, salt, and pepper.

- Bake for between 35-40 minutes or until the bacon becomes crispy. You can also broil the bacon on top if needed.

- Serve with some nice creamed spinach

Avocado Tuna Melt Bites (12 pieces)

Nutrient intake per serving; Carbs: 0.8g, Fat: 11.8g, Protein: 6.2g, Calories: 135

The crispy outside combines with the soft creamy filling on the inside to make a wonderfully tasty dish.

Ingredients

· 10 oz. canned and drained tuna

· A quarter cup of mayonnaise

· A cubed medium avocado

· A quarter cup of parmesan cheese

· A third of a cup of almond flour

· Half a teaspoon of garlic powder

· A quarter teaspoon of onion powder

· Salt and pepper

· Half a cup of coconut oil for frying

How to prepare

· Drain a can of tuna and add to a large sized container where everything will be mixed

· Add mayonnaise, parmesan cheese and spices to the tuna and mix well

- Slice the avocado in half and cube it

- Add avocado into the tuna mixture and fold together. Try not to mash the avocado into the mixture

- Form the tuna mixture into balls and roll into almond flour, covering them completely. Set aside

- Heat the coconut oil in a pan over medium heat. As soon as it's hot, add the tuna balls and fry until all sides are crisp

- Remove from the pan and serve

Bacon, avocado and chicken sandwich (2 servings)

Nutrient intake per serving; Carbs: 2g, Fat: 28.3g, Protein: 22g, Calories: 361

Ingredients

Keto cloud bread

- 3 large eggs

- 3 oz. cream cheese

- An eighth of a teaspoon cream of tartar

- A quarter teaspoon of salt

- Half a teaspoon of garlic powder

Filling

- A tablespoon of mayonnaise

- A teaspoon of siracha

- Two bacon slices

- 3 oz. chicken

- Two pepper jack cheese slices

- 2 grape tomatoes

- A quarter medium avocado

Method of preparation

- Preheat the oven to 300F. Start by separating 3 eggs into two clean dry bowls.

- Add the cream of tartar and salt to the egg whites. Use an electric mixer to whip the whites until they become soft and foamy.

- In a separate bowl, mix 3 oz. of cubed cream cheese with the egg yolks and beat until they become pale yellow

- Gently fold the egg whites into the yolks, half at a time

- On a parchment paper lined baking sheet, spoon 1/4 cup of the keto cloud bread batter.

·   Use a spatula to gently press the tops of the keto cloud bread to form squares. You then sprinkle the tops with garlic powder and bake for about 25 minutes

·   As the keto cloud bread is baking, cook the chicken and bacon with salt and pepper

·   You arrange the sandwich by combining mayo and sriracha and spreading it on the underside of one keto cloud bread. Add the chicken into the mayo mixture.

·   Add the two slices of pepper jack cheese and the bacon. Nestle some halved grape tomatoes and spread the mashed avocado on top. Season to taste and top with the other keto cloud bread.

Crispy Tofu and Bok Choy Salad (3 servings)

Nutrient intake per serving; Carbs: 5.7g, Fat: 35g, Protein: 5g, Calories: 442

Tofu that is baked is quite delicious. You get a rich cube that is full of flavor and crunchy on the outside. Furthermore, raw bok choy is fantastic. It is crunchy and offers a distinct taste to the salad.

Ingredients

Oven baked tofu

·   15 oz. extra firm tofu

- A tablespoon of soy sauce

- A tablespoon of sesame oil

- A tablespoon of water

- Two teaspoons of minced garlic

- A tablespoon of rice wine vinegar

- Juice made from half a lemon

Bok choy salad

- 9 oz. bok choy

- A stalk of green onion

- Two tablespoons of chopped cilantro

- Three tablespoons of coconut oil

- Two tablespoons of soy sauce

- A tablespoon of sambal olek

- A tablespoon of peanut butter

- Juice from half a lime

- Seven drops of liquid stevia

How to prepare

- Begin by pressing the tofu. Place the tofu in a kitchen towel and put something heavy over it. It takes about 4-6 hours to dry out. You may need to change the kitchen towel when halfway done.

·   After pressing the tofu, work on the marinade. Mix all the ingredients for the marinade; soy sauce, sesame oil, water, garlic, vinegar and lemon

·   Chop the tofu into squares and place them in a plastic bag together with the marinade. Let it marinate for at least half an hour. However, overnight is preferred if you can plan for it.

·   Preheat the oven to 350 F. Place the tofu on a baking sheet lined with parchment paper. Bake for half an hour.

·   When the tofu is cooked, start on the bok choy salad. Chop the cilantro and spring onion

·   You then mix all the other ingredients together apart from lime juice and bok choy. You then add cilantro and the spring onion. You can also microwave the coconut oil for about ten seconds so that it melts

·   When the tofu is almost cooked, add the lime juice into the salad dressing and mix together.

·   Chop the bok choy into small pieces.

Remove the tofu from the oven and assemble the salad with tofu, bok choy, and sauce

DINNER RECIPES

Low carb walnut crusted salmon (2 servings)

Nutrient intake per serving; Carbs: 3g, Fat: 43g, Protein: 20g, Calories: 373

In the ketogenic diet, fatty fish is proven to lower cholesterol and aids with your overall health. This recipe is easy to prepare and super tasty. It takes under 15 minutes to prepare.

Ingredients

· Half a cup of walnuts

· Two tablespoons of sugar-free maple syrup

· Half a tablespoon of Dijon mustard

· A quarter teaspoon of dill

· Two, 3oz. salmon fillets

· A tablespoon of olive oil

· Salt and pepper

How to prepare

· Preheat the oven to 350F. Add half a cup of walnuts to the food processor

· Add two tablespoons of maple syrup and your spices

- Add a tablespoon of mustard

- Pulse this in the food processor until paste-like

- Heat a pan or skillet with a tablespoon of oil until very hot. Thoroughly dry the salmon fillets and place them skin down in the pan. Let it sear for about 3 minutes, undisturbed.

- As it sears, add the walnut mixture to the top side of the salmon fillets

- After that, transfer them to an oven and bake for about 8 minutes

- Serve with fresh spinach, enjoy. You can sprinkle a little bit of smoked paprika on top.

Keto Hot Chili Soup (4 servings)

Nutrient intake per serving; Carbs: 5.8g, Fat: 27.8g, Protein: 28g, Calories: 396

Ingredients

- A teaspoon of coriander seeds

- Two tablespoons of olive oil

- Two sliced chili peppers

- Two cups of chicken broth

- Two cups of water

- A teaspoon of turmeric

- Half a teaspoon of ground cumin

- Four tablespoons of tomato paste

- 16 oz. chicken thighs

- Two tablespoons of butter

- A medium avocado

- 2 oz. queso fresco

- Four tablespoons of fresh chopped cilantro

- Juice from half a lime

- Salt and pepper

How to prepare

- Cut and set the chicken thighs to cook in an oiled pan. Season it with salt and pepper. You then leave it aside.

- Heat up the coriander seeds to release more flavor with two tablespoons of olive oil

- Once they are fragrant, add in the sliced chili peppers to add their flavor to the oil

- You then add in the broth and water. Let it simmer and season. Add turmeric, ground cumin, salt and pepper to taste

- As the soup simmers, add in the tomato paste and butter. Stir so that it melts and mixes. Let the soup simmer for between 5-10 minutes.

- Lower the heat on the stove and add the juice from half the lime

- Place 4oz of chicken thighs into the bottom of the bowl so that you can pour soup over it.

- Ladle the soup for serving. Garnish with a quarter of an avocado into each bowl, half an ounce of queso fresco and cilantro

Slow-Cooker Ketogenic Chicken Tikka Masala (5 servings)

Nutrient intake per serving; Carbs: 5.8g, Fat: 41.2g, Protein: 26g, Calories: 493

Ingredients

- One ½ lbs. chicken thighs, bone-in-skin-on

- 1 lb. chicken thighs, boneless, skinless

- Two tablespoons of olive oil

- Two teaspoons of onion powder

- Three cloves of minced garlic

- An inch of grated ginger root

- 3 tablespoons of tomato paste

- 5 teaspoons of garam masala

- 2 teaspoons of smoked paprika

- 4 teaspoons of kosher salt

- 10 oz can of diced tomatoes

- A cup of heavy cream

- A cup of coconut milk

- Fresh chopped cilantro

- A teaspoon of guar gum

How to prepare

- De-bone the chicken on the bone-in chicken thighs. Chop all the chicken pieces into bite-sized pieces. Ensure that you keep the skin for the pieces that have it.

- Add the chicken to a slow cooker and grate an inch of ginger over the top

- Add all the dry spices into the slow cooker and mix properly

·   Add canned diced tomatoes and tomato paste into the slow cooker and mix well

·   Finally, add half a cup of coconut milk and mix well. Cook over low heat for 6 hours or 3 hours over high heat.

·   Once the slow-cooking is over, add the remainder of the coconut milk, heavy cream, and guar gum and mix well into the chicken. This will help the curry thicken nicely.

·   Serve over cauliflower rice or a veggie of your choice

Barbeque Bacon Cheeseburger Waffles (2 servings)

Nutrient intake per serving; Carbs: 3g, Fat: 29.8g, Protein: 18.8g, Calories: 354

This meal is dense with calories, delicious, and it's best to have when you know you will have an active day.

Ingredients

Waffles

·   5 oz. of cheddar cheese

·   Two large eggs

·   A cup of cauliflower crumbles

- A quarter teaspoon of garlic powder

- A quarter teaspoon of onion powder

- Four tablespoons of almond flour

- Three tablespoons of parmesan cheese

- Salt and pepper

The topping

- 4 oz. ground beef

- Four slices of chopped bacon

- Four tablespoons of sugar-free barbeque sauce

- 1.5 oz. of cheddar cheese

- Salt and pepper

How to prepare

- Shred 3 oz. of cheese. You will use half for the waffle and half on top.

- Measure out the cauliflower crumbles over a scale, or use a cup

- Mix in half of the cheddar cheese, parmesan cheese, eggs, almond flour, and spices

- Slice the bacon thin over medium to high heat

- As soon as the bacon is partially cooked, add in the beef.

- Add any excess grease from the pan into the waffle mixture that you set aside

- Immersion blend the waffle mixture into a paste that is thick

- Add half the mixture to the waffle iron and cook until crisp. Repeat for the second waffle

- As the waffles cook, add the sugar-free BBQ sauce to the bacon and ground beef mixture.

- Assemble the waffles by adding half of the ground beef mixture and half of the remaining cheddar cheese to the top of the waffle

- Broil for about two minutes until the cheese is nicely melted over the top

- Serve immediately. You may want to slice up a green onion to sprinkle over the top.

Bacon Cheeseburger Casserole (6 servings)

Nutrient intake per serving; Carbs: 3.6g, Fat: 35.5g, Protein: 32.2g, Calories: 478

Ingredients

- 1 lb. ground beef

- Three slices of bacon

- Half a cup of almond flour

- 256g of cauliflower, riced

- A tablespoon of psyllium husk powder

- Half a teaspoon of garlic powder

- Half a teaspoon of onion powder

- Two tablespoons of reduced sugar ketchup

- A tablespoon of Dijon mustard

- Two tablespoons of mayonnaise

- Three large eggs

- 4 oz. cheddar cheese

- Salt and pepper

How to prepare

- Preheat the oven to 350F. Put rice cauliflower in the food processor and add dry ingredients. Mix well

- Put bacon and ground beef in a food processor until crumbly. Cook over medium to high heat. Season with salt and pepper

· Shred the cheese as the meat cooks. Once the meat is done, mix all the ingredients in a large bowl and add half of the cheddar cheese.

· Add eggs, mayo, ketchup and mustard to the mixture. Use a fork or hands to mix everything well

· Press the mixture into a 9x9 baking pan lined with parchment paper. You then top with the other half of the cheddar cheese

· Place on the top rack of the oven and bake for 25-30 minutes. For additional crisp on top, broil for around 3 minutes or until browned

· Remove from oven and let it cool for 5 to 10 minutes

· Slice and serve with additional toppings

DESSERT RECIPES

Pumpkin Pecan Pie Ice Cream (4 one cup servings)

Nutrient intake per serving; Carbs: 4.3g, Fat: 22.3g, Protein: 6.5g, Calories: 248

For extra decadence, you can add 3-4 oz. of cream cheese to this recipe. This recipe requires an iced cream maker.

Ingredients

- Half a cup of cottage cheese

- Half a cup of pumpkin puree

- A teaspoon of pumpkin spice

- Two cups of coconut milk

- Half a teaspoon of xantham gum

- Three large egg yolks

- A third of a cup erythritol

- 20 drops of liquid stevia

- A teaspoon of maple extract

- Half a cup of pecans that are toasted and chopped

- Two tablespoons of salted butter

How to prepare

- Chop the toasted pecans and put on the stove with butter. Leave it over low heat until the butter turns brown. In case you don't have toasted pecans, place in a pan and toast over low heat for between 7-10 minutes

- Place all the ingredients into a container that can accommodate the immersion blender

·   Use your immersion blender to blend all the ingredients together into a mixture that is smooth

·   Add the mixture to your ice cream machine

·   Once your butter turns brown and the pecans have soaked up some of the butter, place it inside the ice cream machine

·   Follow the churning instructions as per your ice cream manufacturer's instructions

Ketogenic Amaretti Cookies (16 cookies)

Nutrient intake per serving; Carbs: 1.2g, Fat: 7.9g, Protein: 2.4g, Calories: 86

These cookies are delicate and sweet. Each one is soft and full of almond and fruity flavors. This recipe uses strawberry jam, but you could swap it out for other jams.

Ingredients

·   A cup of almond flour

·   Two tablespoons of coconut flour

·   Half a teaspoon of baking powder

·   A quarter teaspoon of baking powder

·   A quarter teaspoon of cinnamon

- Half a teaspoon of salt

- Half a cup of erythritol

- Two large eggs

- Four tablespoons of coconut oil

- Half a teaspoon of vanilla extract

- Half a teaspoon of almond extract

- Two tablespoons of sugar-free jam

- One tablespoon of organic shredded coconut

How to prepare

- Preheat the oven to 350F. mix all the dry ingredients and whisk.

- Add in the wet ingredients and mix well. Use a whisk or hand mixer.

- Form the cookies on a parchment paper-lined baking sheet. Add an indent at the middle of each cookie using your finger or the back of a measuring spoon.

- Bake for about 15 minutes or until the cookies turn golden or crack slightly.

- Let the cookies cool on a wire rack and fill each indent with sugar-free jam

- Lastly, sprinkle some shredded coconut on top of each cookie

- Dish out and serve

No Bake Coconut Cashew Bars (8 servings)

Nutrient intake per serving; Carbs: 4g, Fat: 17.6g, Protein: 4g, Calories: 189

These bars are easy to make and can be frozen or refrigerated depending on your needs.

Ingredients

- A cup of almond flour

- A quarter cup of melted butter

- A quarter cup of sugar-free maple syrup

- A teaspoon of cinnamon

- A pinch of salt

- Half a cup of cashews

- A quarter cup of shredded coconut

How to prepare

·   Mix the melted butter and almond flour in a large bowl

·   Add cinnamon, salt, and sugar-free maple syrup and mix properly

·   You then add the shredded coconut and mix again

·   Roughly chop half a cup of cashews whether raw or roasted. Add to the coconut cashew bar dough. Mix well

·   Line a baking dish with parchment paper and spread the coconut cashew bar dough in an even layer. You can add some more shredded coconut and cinnamon on top

·   Place them in the refrigerator and chill for at least two hours. However, overnight is recommended. As soon as they are chilled, slice them into bars. Serve and enjoy!

Ketogenic Chocolate Covered macaroons (12 macaroons)

Nutrient intake per serving; Carbs: 1g, Fat: 7.3g, Protein: 1g, Calories: 73

These macaroons are sweet with nice coconut, almond, and chocolate flavors.

Ingredients

- A cup of unsweetened shredded coconut

- A large white egg

- A quarter cup of erythritol

- Half a teaspoon of almond extract

- A pinch of salt

- 20 grams of sugar-free chocolate

- Two tablespoons of coconut oil

How to prepare

- Preheat the oven to 350 F and spread a cup of shredded and unsweetened coconut into a thin layer on a parchment paper-lined baking sheet. As soon as the oven is hot enough, place the coconut in to toast a little for about five minutes.

- As the coconut toasts, beat the egg white until it's foamy

- Add the erythritol and a pinch of salt as you continue to mix.

- You then add the almond extract for a twist on normal coconut macaroons.

- Once the coconut flakes have toasted and cooled, add them into the mix and fold everything together

·   Use an ice cream scoop or your hands to tightly pack little balls of macaroon batter and gently place them on a parchment paper-lined baking sheet. Bake until they are golden. This should take around 15 minutes.

·   As they bake, make the chocolate drizzle by melting coconut oil and the sugar-free chocolate. Continuously stir to make sure the chocolate doesn't burn.

·   When the macaroons are out of the oven, drizzle your chocolate over each one of them.

Ketogenic Chocolate Peanut Butter Tarts (4 servings)

Nutrient intake per serving; Carbs: 3.9g, Fat: 26.8g, Protein: 9.8g, Calories:305

Ingredients

Crust

·   A quarter cup of flaxseeds

·   Two tablespoons of almond flour

·   A tablespoon of erythritol

·   A large egg white

Top layer

·   A medium avocado

- Four tablespoons of cocoa powder

- A quarter cup of erythritol

- Half a teaspoon of vanilla extract

- Half a teaspoon of cinnamon

- Two tablespoons of heavy cream

Middle layer

- Four tablespoons of peanut butter

- Two tablespoons of butter

How to prepare

- Preheat the oven to 350 F. Make your crust by grinding up a quarter cup of flax seeds until they are finely ground.

- Add the rest of the crust ingredients to the ground flaxseeds. Blend until well mixed

- Press the crust mixture into the tart pans and up the sides. Bake for 8 minutes until set

- As the crust bakes, prepare the top layer by mixing all the ingredients in a blender and blend until smooth and creamy

- After removing the crusts from the oven, let them cool as you prepare your peanut butter layer. Melt the peanut butter and butter in the microwave or a small pan over the stove until well mixed and soft

·   Pour the melted layer of peanut butter onto the tart crusts and place in the fridge for half an hour until set

·   As soon as the top of the peanut butter layer is set, add the chocolate avocado layer on top. Smooth it out and refrigerate for an hour.

·   Slice, serve and enjoy

Ketogenic bodybuilding meal plans for men /women

If you're trying to gain muscle mass while losing weight, here are examples of how your meals should break down:

Men

Nutrient intake per serving:

- Carbs: 2
- Fat: 36.3
- Protein: 44.2
- Calories: 521

Breakfast

- Four eggs

- An ounce of cheddar cheese

- Four bacon slices

Pre-workout shake

Nutrient intake per serving; Carbs: 9.3, Fat: 18.6, Protein: 31g, Calories: 318

- A scoop of whey

- 250ml of unsweetened almond milk

- Two tablespoons of peanut butter

Lunch

Nutrient intake per serving; Carbs: 14.3, Fat: 26.7, Protein: 49.8, Calories: 503

- 200g of chicken breast trimmed of fat / 200g turkey breasts/ 220g tilapia

- Side salad (60g spinach, half a carrot, half a cucumber and a stalk of celery

- 50g avocado

- Two tablespoons of balsamic vinegar

- A tablespoon of olive oil

Dinner

Nutrient intake per serving; Carbs: 9.9, Fat: 15, Protein: 55.2, Calories: 389

- 150g veggies

- A tablespoon of butter

Snack

Nutrient intake per serving; Carbs: 14.5, Fat: 19.7g, Protein: 23.6g, Calories: 324

- 200g of 4% cottage cheese

- 20 almonds or peanuts

Women

Breakfast

Nutrient intake per serving; Carb: 1.2g, Fat: 24.6g, Protein: 28.6g, Calories: 347

- Two eggs

- An ounce of cheddar cheese

- Three bacon slices

Post workout

Nutrient intake per serving; Carbs: 17g, Fat: 10.6, Protein: 27g, Calories: 268

- A scoop of whey

- A cup of unsweetened almond milk

- A cup of strawberries/almond butter

Lunch

Nutrient intake per serving; Carbs: 15.8g, Fat: 21.1g, Protein: 51.1g, Calories- 462

- 7 ounces of chicken breasts trimmed of fat

- Salad (two cups of spinach, half a carrot, half a cucumber, and half a tomato)

- Two ounces of feta cheese

- Two tablespoons of balsamic vinegar

- A tablespoon of olive oil

Snack

Nutrient intake per serving; Carbs: 5.2g, Fat: 12g, Protein: 5.1g, Calories: 139

- 20 almonds or peanuts

Dinner

Nutrient intake per serving; Carbs: 12.2g, Fat: 19.9g, Protein: 49.6g, Calories: 426

- 7 ounces sirloin trimmed of fat

- 6 ounces veggies

· A tablespoon of butter

The Right Way of Cooking Vegetables

There are cooking methods that preserve nutrients in veggies while others can destroy them.

· Limit your water use

When veggies are cooked in water, they lose nutrients. To retain the nutrients, cook veggies in as little water as possible for the minimal amount of time. Steaming and microwaving also lead to less loss of nutrients.

· Use some fat

Veggie nutrients like beta-carotene, vitamin D and K are fat-soluble and can only enter the bloodstream with some fat.

· Wash before cutting

Cutting veggies allow the escape of nutrients. By washing prior to cutting, nutrients will safely remain in the cell walls.

· Keep the vegetable peels on if possible

Chapter Summary

- This chapter was your personal keto cookbook and contained recipes for breakfast, lunch, dinner, and dessert.
- We also gave a sample of types of foods to eat if you want to gain muscle.

In the next chapter, you will learn tips on how to be successful on the Ketogenic diet.

Chapter Eleven: Ketogenic Diet Success Tips

Foods to Avoid With the Ketogenic Diet

In the last chapter we gave you many handy recipes to use while on the Ketogenic Diet. You'll notice some ingredients that are probably part of your regular menu were nowhere to be found. That's because there are some foods you must stay away from on the Keto Diet. Any foods that are high in carbohydrates should be limited. You should cut down on sugary foods, grains or starches, fruits, beans, root veggies and tubers, low fat items (due to high sugar content), selected sauces, booze and completely sugar free diets.

1. French fries and potato chips

French fries and potato chips are fattening and unhealthy. These fried potatoes contain a lot of calories and you can consume a lot of them in one sitting. Consumption of fries and potato chips is connected to gaining weight. A study revealed that these foods contribute to weight gain more than any other food. Furthermore, baked, roasted or fried potatoes contain cancer-causing ingredients. When you do eat them, it is advisable to eat plain, boiled potatoes.

2. Drinks that are sugary

Beverages like soda are one of the unhealthiest things on earth. They are strongly linked to gaining of weight and are detrimental to your health if drunk in excess. Liquid calories do not make you feel satisfied and you will add these calories on top of your normal daily calorie count. If you want to lose weight, steer clear of these drinks.

3. White bread

It is highly refined and contains lots of added sugars. It ranks high on the glycemic index and can raise levels of sugar. A study revealed that eating two slices of white bread in a day was linked to a greater risk of gaining weight and becoming obese. Bread that is made from very fine flour can raise sugar levels and cause one to overeat.

4. Candy bars

They are quite unhealthy because they stack a lot of sugar, added oils, and refined flour. Furthermore, they are high in calories and low in nutrition value. An regular candy bar contains an average of 250 calories. If you are craving snacks, eat a fruit or nuts.

5. Most fruit juices

Many of the fruit juices found in stores have very little similarity to a whole fruit. They are highly processed and contain a lot of sugar. They contain as much sugar as soda, sometimes even more. These juices also contain no fiber so they will not have the same effect as real fruits.

6. Pastries and cakes

These have unhealthy ingredients such as added sugar and refined flour. They also contain artificial Trans-fats which are very harmful and connected to several diseases.

Additionally, they aren't satisfying meaning you will feel hungry very fast after eating them and are likely to eat more.

7. Alcohol

It provides more calories than carbohydrates and protein. Consumption of alcohol in moderation is okay; however, heavy drinking is linked to excessive weight gain. Beer is especially fattening but even liquor tends to have a high sugar content.

8. Ice cream

This is quite unhealthy, high in calories and loaded with sugar. Think about making your own ice cream using less sugar and healthier ingredients like yogurt and fruit. If you are going to have it, serve yourself small portions to avoid eating too much.

9. Pizza

Ones that are made commercially are very unhealthy. They contain high calories and often contain unhealthy ingredients such as refined flour and meat that is processed. Many popular chains tend to use sauces that are high in sugar too. It is better to make pizzas at home so you can use fresh, unrefined ingredients..

10. Coffee drinks with high calories

Specialty drinks from coffee chains can be loaded with empty calories that can equal a whole meal. Sugary, milky, drinks like a frappuccino, have artificial ingredients that are very unhealthy and fattening. However, plain, black coffee is very healthy and can aid in fat burning.

11. Foods with a lot of added sugar

This speaks for itself. Some examples are sugary breakfast cereals, packaged items, some 'nutrition' bars (many have a lot of added sugar, be sure to read labels), and flavored yogurt.

12. Soy sauce

Even though it is low on calories, it has a high sodium content that can make you bloated and increase your chances of getting hypertension.

13. Tropical fruits

There are some to avoid if you want to lose weight. Have limited mangoes and ripe pineapples because they contain a lot of sugar.

Foods You Should Eat

You should consume plenty of meat, fatty fish, eggs, butter and cream, cheese, nuts and seeds, healthy oils, avocados, low carb veggies, and condiments.

In case you feel like eating something between meals, the following are advised for snacking:

- Fatty fish or meat
- Cheese

- A handful of nuts
- Cheese with olives
- 1-2 hard-boiled eggs
- 90% dark chocolate

Tips for Eating Out on a Ketogenic Diet

Restaurants usually offer some kind of meat or fish or dishes that are fish based. You can order this and replace foods containing high carbs with veggies. Meals that are egg-based are also a good idea. In short, when eating out, choose meat, fish or egg-based foods. Also, order extra vegetables rather than carbohydrates or starch.

Supplements for a Ketogenic Diet

Even though taking supplements is not needed, some could prove helpful.

- MCT oil- it is added to drinks or yogurt. It gives energy and aids in the increment of ketone levels.
- Minerals- added salt and other minerals are useful when beginning the diet. This is because of the alterations in mineral and water balance.
- Caffeine- can provide energy, aid in losing fat, and enhance performance
- Exogenous ketones- this supplement can help in raising the levels of ketones in the body
- Creatine- this supplement has several benefits for one's health and performance. It is advisable if one combines ketogenic diets with exercise.
- Whey- this increases your daily protein intake.

Commonly Asked Questions About the Ketogenic Diet

- Can I ever eat carbohydrates again?

Yes, you can, even though it is advisable to get rid of them when starting. After sixty to ninety days, you can eat carbs once in a while.

- Will I lose muscles?

In any weight loss diet, the risk of losing muscles exists. However, with the ketogenic diet, you reduce the chances of muscle loss, especially if you lift weights and use the protein supplements.

- Can this diet aid in building muscle?

Yes, it can. However, it may not be as effective as a moderate carb diet plan.

- Do I ever need to load carbs?

Nope, although a few days with high-calorie foods may be beneficial, especially before activity.

- How much protein is one required to eat?

The quantity of protein has to be moderate because very high amounts can raise the levels of insulin and actually lower ketones. A maximum of 35% of the total calorie intake should be protein.

- How do I deal with fatigue?

Lower the intake of carbs and refer to the above tips.

- Why do my urine and breath smell?

Urine smell is due to the removal of by-products created during ketosis. For fresh breath, chew some sugar-free gum or drink naturally flavored water.

Chapter Summary

This chapter was about:

- Foods to avoid when on the Ketogenic diet
- Frequently Asked Questions

In the last chapter, you will learn how to combine both the intermittent and ketogenic diets.

Chapter Twelve: Combining Intermittent Fasting and Ketogenic Diets

You may be asking yourself whether you can combine the two diets to aid in your weight loss. Well, we are going to discuss how you can blend the two for perfect health. These are the most practiced diets at the moment because of their massive benefits- and you can follow both of them at the same time. Not only are they compatible, but these two diets also complement each other.

If you are set on combining these two diet plans, I will offer some tips that will assist you in succeeding.

Please make sure that you still consume enough food. Intermittent fasting will naturally aid you in eating less during the day but you still need to ensure that you are eating nutritious keto meals to keep any deficiencies or metabolic problems at bay. Make use of an app or website to know the correct calorie and macro intake on a daily basis.

How Intermittent Fasting Complements the Keto Diet

1.   It will make you go into ketosis much faster

One of the basic goals of the keto diet is to get into ketosis as fast as possible and to stick there for the longest period. When you are intermittently fasting, the state of fasting will starve your body for carbs. This means that your sugar levels will drop much more compared to a person who is not fasting. As a result, your body will resort to burning your fat reserves and ketones much faster. Consequently, you will get into ketosis faster.

When you are in ketosis, it's like you are fasting because your body will generate fuel by burning it's fat. If you have been on an intermittent fasting diet but there are no positive results yet, you can embark on the keto diet during your eating window. You will notice positive changes as well as great results.

2.   Fast weight loss

Both diet plans are designed to make your body shift from burning glucose to burning fat. Your fat burning is optimized when you combine both diets. The reason is this: as soon as the keto diet has put you into ketosis, your body will already be adapted to burning fat for fuel. So, when you add the intermittent fasting plan, your body will already be used to fat burning and will continue being effective in burning fat for fuel. You can compare this to a person who doesn't follow the ketogenic diet. When they start on intermittent fasting, their bodies will be slow in entering the fasted phase where all the fat burning occurs.

3.   Improved brain health and boosted mental focus

Our brains are the body's greatest consumers of energy. It's also a fact that fat is the most energy efficient fuel compared to glucose. Intermittent fasting and the keto diet make the body burn fat for fuel and this is quite beneficial to our brain health. We always have stored fat that is available to be converted to energy and so, provided your body is trained to burn fat for fuel, your brain will always have a constant supply of energy. This is the exact reason why those who follow both the intermittent and keto plans see more mental focus, clarity, and unrivaled neurological gains.

That's not all, several studies have also revealed that fasting promotes the production of BDNF, a protein that nurtures the brain stem cells and boosts mental health.

4.   The two diets become easier

Honestly, one of the major reasons most of us are afraid of intermittent fasting is because it leaves us feeling starved. On the other hand, the keto diet is proven to aid in lowering hunger and cravings because of the high-fat content in the diet plan. If you are already on the ketogenic diet regime, you will find it easier to manage the fasting window when on an intermittent fasting plan. The two diet plans are tailored to maintain insulin levels, resulting in reduced hunger and cravings.

5.   Improved exercise

You may ask yourself whether it's possible to exercise while fasting. Far from being recommended, research studies have also revealed that being on both the keto and intermittent diet plans will boost the long-term gains of an exercise regime. These two diet plans train the body to burn fat for fuel and this triggers metabolic changes that boost one's workout performance when fasting.

Furthermore, you will also gain muscle as you train on a fasting plan. Studies done on Muslim athletes who fast during Ramadan have shown no negative effects on performance. It is also proven that when you do strength training while fasting, what you eat after will be better used by your body as compared to when you are not fasting.

10 Tips for Starting and Sticking With the Two Diet Plans

1. Monitor your body

Just like with any new diet or exercise plan, only you will know what works for you. Everybody is unique and will respond differently to the same diet plans. If you are on the 16/8 intermittent fasting plan but you realize that you are struggling, don't be afraid to make changes. Try to move your eating window later in the day or make sure that you are eating enough high-quality keto foods.

2. Don't start both eating plans at the same time

Even if you are very excited about getting on both diet plans, if you are new to them, it is not advisable for you to embark on both of them at the same time. Attempting to master the ketogenic diet as well as sticking to the intermittent fasting plan can take a toll on you and you will most likely throw in the towel early.

I would advise that you start on the intermittent fasting plan for about fourteen days to allow your body to adjust to the new diet. As a result, your body will be more adept to shifting to it's fat burning phase, so when you start on the ketogenic diet plan, you will get into ketosis much faster.

3. Drink tea

You are allowed to have as much calorie-free beverages during the fasting window as you'd like. Tea is greatly recommended to keep you hydrated as it also boosts gut health, keeps cravings at bay, and aids in detoxification of the body.

4. Focus on the food

Even though keto and intermittent fasting reduce your appetite as well as cravings, be sure you choose the right meals. Keep in mind that you don't want to overdo it with the protein; cook with some healthy fats to boost your energy.

5. Increase your water drinking

Whether you are on a diet or not, water is important and a must-have. Water helps you to get full faster and avoid overeating. You can also add keto-friendly foods like cucumber to your drinking water if you'd like some flavor.

6. Steer clear of sugar-free drinks

A majority of people assume that having sugar-free drinks is okay, but the truth is that the wrong artificial sugar can sabotage your diet plan. Avoid diet soda, flavored water, or energy drinks.

7. Keep yourself busy

Having a lot of free time on your hands will make you want to snack. You need to occupy yourself with activities such as exercise, movies, or reading.

8. Come up with a sleeping routine

Having a regular sleeping pattern is important. The right amount of sleep will definitely impact your eating habits and mood. It is easier if you fast through your sleeping time. If you are up all hours you'll feel the need to eat again.

9. Manage your stress

Allowing yourself to be stressed will definitely trigger overeating, which will make it impossible to maintain your intermittent fasting plan. Stress can make you focus on eating unhealthy foods to make yourself feel better. Therefore, learn to control your stress levels while on a diet.

10. The major hurdle is your own motivation

There is always a mental obstruction to get over. You will may worry that the diet plans will affect your thinking, whether you will black out, if you'll fail, and so forth. The truth is you just need to be mindful and get through it, and you'll be fine.

Ketogenic and Intermittent Fasting Boosts Sports Performance

Top athletes have confessed that these two diet plans have helped increase their athletic performance. In case your goal is to improve your sports performance, these two diets are the remedy. Since they train the body to burn fat, they help one recover from exercise much faster. The easier it is for the body to burn fat, the better your performance and recovery time.

Self-Healing of the Body

Intermittent fasting leads to autophagy in the body. This means that it eats up its own cells and tissues for the better. What autophagy essentially does is get rid of harmful and toxic elements in the cells and recycle damaged proteins. Autophagy takes place when the body is starved and when proteins and carbs are limited. All of this happens in the intermittent and keto diet plans. Blending these two diet plans enable us to reap the benefits efficiently, and in a healthy manner.

Cons of the Intermittent Fasting Diet Plan

1. Disruption of social eating

Eating is a social activity. Most celebrations and special occasions revolve around meals together with the people we adore. Since this diet plan is quite different from the traditional patterns of eating for most people, it may get in the way of your social gatherings.

You may find it difficult to be at social gatherings where there is a lot of drinking and eating. Additionally, you may also find it difficult to attend dinners or even lunch meetings.

2. Hunger and low energy

Since we are used to snacking or having meals throughout the day, when that changes, we might be left feeling hungry and less productive. A few studies have revealed that intermittent fasting may cause constipation, feeling cold, short tempers and even reduced concentration. One may not even feel the motivation to be involved in physical activity. However, other studies disagree and say that the diet does not dwarf one's ability to work out.

3. Binge eating

During the feeding windows, some people may take this chance to consume excessive calories. It is very normal to begin binge eating after a period of fasting.

4. Digestion problems

Several people may face problems with digestion when large amounts of food are consumed within a short duration of time. Larger quantities of food mean that they need more time to be digested, and this causes additional stress which leads to bloating and indigestion. This can have huge implications especially for those who already have gastrointestinal issues. This is the reason why people who suffer from digestive issues are advised to eat regularly and avoid skipping meals.

5. Not everyone can get on this diet

If you have a medical condition, it is advisable not to start on this diet because it may have negative effects on your overall health. For example, people suffering from diabetes or hypoglycemia require glucose all through the day and going without it can be very risky. You should also know that if you have ever had a history of eating disorders, then intermittent fasting is not recommended for you.

6. Long-term health implications

When this diet is taken too far, there is always a risk of deficiencies and abnormalities that will have an effect on fertility as well as reproduction in women. Intermittent fasting is linked to fertility and menopause in women. As per studies conducted on animals, fasting resulted in decreased body weight, blood sugar levels, as well as reduced ovary size.

Fasting can disrupt the levels of the luteinizing hormones, estradiol, and ghrelin, which influence appetite as well as reproduction. In the year 2017, a research study involving women revealed that three days of absolute fasting during the mid-follicular phases influenced the luteinizing hormone but did not affect the follicle development or the menstrual cycle.

A different study also revealed that overweight women experienced longer menstrual cycles after intermittent fasting as compared to those who were undergoing continuous energy restriction.

Chapter Summary

- Combining Intermittent Fasting and the Ketogenic Diet
- Tips, Pros of combining the two diets, and cons

Final Thoughts

Intermittent fasting will have very good results if done right. If you have been thinking of getting on an intermittent fasting regime, then it is time to do so. Simply follow the steps discussed in this guide, taking care to choose a plan that works for you depending on your lifestyle and how your days are planned out.

Start small, take the fast one day at a time, and feed well, ensuring that you nourish your body with the right nutrients. As you go along, you can add some exercises to your daily plan to get the most out of it.

Change up different areas of these diets to customize them to your needs. Make it more of your own plan so that it works better for you. Lastly, avoid the common mistakes we've talked about in this book.

Intermittent fasting doesn□'t have to be a hassle. It can be done in a way that is natural and easy, as we have seen throughout this book.

You can feel at ease having addressed all your fears of fasting and begin the journey to becoming a better, hopefully, leaner, and definitely healthier version of yourself. There'□s no need to wait anymore. Go ahead, start fasting and enjoy good food- especially by using the Keto recipes in this book- while you□'re at it.

This book has given you the proven steps and strategies on how to get into a ketogenic diet that is easy and beneficial to your health.

The Ketogenic diet is one of the most popular diets in the world of weight loss right now for many reasons. Thousands have enjoyed the many health benefits including lower blood pressure, lower cholesterol, more energy, clearer thinking, and, of course, weight loss. Many also believe that the ketogenic diet can even help fight cancer.

The ketogenic diet allows you to eat real foods, the ones you are already used to eating, and you will still lose the weight you want to lose. Using proven methods to help your body and metabolism work together, you will lose weight and build muscles in your sleep!

Now that you know the Intermittent Fasting and Ketogenic Diet basics it is time to put what you have read into practice. You have the recipes, benefits, tools, and proven ways of benefiting from these diets together in your hands. If you follow what you read here, you can easily get started on your healthful journey, customize, and maintain it.

I hope this book was able to help you to eat, live healthily, and achieve all-around wellness by following the Intermittent fasting and Ketogenic diets.

If you enjoyed and found this book valuable, please leave a short review on Amazon!

Made in the USA
Middletown, DE
17 April 2019